THE GREEN ARTE

THE GREEN ARTE
Craft of the Herbwise

Josh Williams

AEON

First published in 2022 by
Aeon Books

Copyright © 2022 by Josh Williams

The right of Josh Williams to be identified as the author of this work has been asserted in accordance with §§ 77 and 78 of the Copyright Design and Patents Act 1988.

All rights reserved. No part of this publication may be reproduced, stored in a retrieval system, or transmitted, in any form or by any means, electronic, mechanical, photocopying, recording, or otherwise, without the prior written permission of the publisher.

British Library Cataloguing in Publication Data

A C.I.P. for this book is available from the British Library

ISBN-13: 978-1-80152-044-7

Cover art by Charlotte Pili, 2021 / @BrambleGhost
Typeset by Medlar Publishing Solutions Pvt Ltd, India
Printed in Great Britain

www.aeonbooks.co.uk

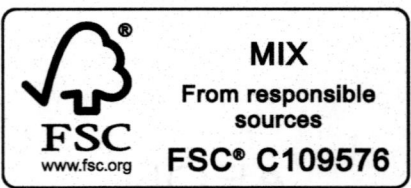

CONTENTS

Invocation	1
A New Map of Ancient Tracks	3
The Green Arte	7
Initiations and The Mysteries	9
The Nature of the Hedgewalker	11
Relationships of Rightness	15
Shrouded in Green	21
Between the Lines	25
The Center of the World	29
The Green Realm	33
Chlorophyll	37
Verdant Breath	41

Vital Force	45
Entering the Green	53
The Green Grammar	59
Kith and Kin	61
Deities of the Green Realm	63
Of River, Mountain, Meadow, and Desert	71
Sacred Circles	77
Ivy in the Skull	81
Garland of the Year	85
Lunar Tides	97
Raising the Hedge	105
A Map to the Green Realm	109
Invoking the Plant Spirits	117
Plant Spirit Dedications	123
The Familiar Green Spirit	133
Sacred Fires	135
Plant Spirit Shrines	139
Plant Spirit Vessels	145
Petitioning the Plant Spirits	151
Plant Medicine	155
Tools of the Arte	161
Medicine, Magic, and Mystery	169
Plant Spirit Magic	173
The Shared Meal	183
The Green Ritual	187
Divination	193
Taboos	199
Stewardship and Sovereignty	205
Shrine and Grove Tending	209
Writing Charms, Petitions, and Rituals	217
The Keep	223
The Wild Within	225
The Plant Priesthood	229
A Grammar of the Green Arte	233
Stay Connected	255
REFERENCES AND RESOURCES	257
INDEX	259

INVOCATION

I call the Great Green God, Verdant Lord, Evergreen King!
You who knows the mysteries of the green realm and guards them well,
   You who take the plant spirits all as your wards,
   You who keep the ancient tracks …

Mighty Green God, who haunts the primordial forest and ushers life into this world, and out of it at its appointed time! Take repast of these offerings laid here in your honor—let them be gifts given for countless gifts received, let them fulfill our bond of sacred reciprocity, let them strengthen our kinship from this world to yours!

Great Verdant One, your dance is the dance of the wild world; it is you who warms the soil and rouses the seeds when the days become bright, calling forth sap and sprout across the whole of the earth. It is you who summons winter slumber and lulls green spirits into their roots when the days become dark. By your wisdom does life emerge from fertile soil, and by it all life is returned to the great cauldron of decay, rot, and compost only to become the ground which nourishes new life in the season to come.

Mighty Green God, whatever work is done with the plant spirits all is done in your domain. You are the great guardian of green mysteries, green spirits, and green spaces. Under your watchful eye the plant spirits all are kept well, and by your blessing alone are their secrets revealed to the seeker.

Great Verdant One, who moves across the hedge, keeper of the gates, knower of secret paths and ancient tracks. Open wide and clear the ways for me that I may travel by a blue-green light into the depths of the ancient woodlands; seeking out the purest wisdom, I wander these tracks and follow your gentle footprints.

Evergreen God of the primordial forest—come, with staff and satchel, as teacher and guide, and bring us into the old ways of the green realm. Make strong our connections to familiar plants, saturate our medicine with magic and our magic with medicine, and with rustling leaves whisper the secrets of the emerald artes into our longing hearts.

Great Green Man, by and by, let us perceive your presence through silence and stealth. Chase away all inauspiciousness from this heart and from this hearth making this a sacred grove filled with your virtues. With honor, accept the gifts of word and deed laid out here before you and make fertile the soil of our spirits that all good will grow here.

A NEW MAP OF ANCIENT TRACKS

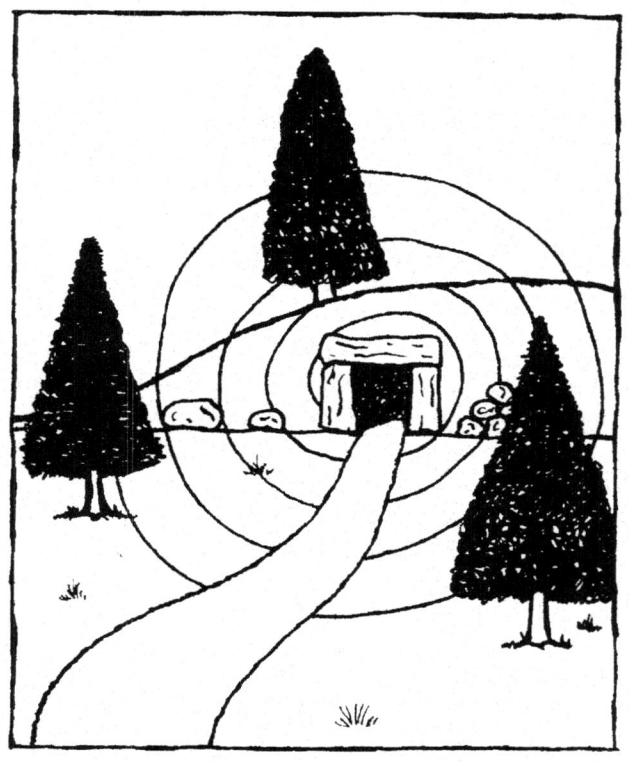

The plants that nourish us in all their countless ways have a secret. What we see of them is what exists above the ground, in our world. But hidden below, in the dark and mysterious and sometimes terrifying depths, are the roots of these beings. These roots reach down into the very subconscious of the world itself, down to where we find our own hazy beginnings: the pitch-black womb. Where these roots touch we aren't always sure. We can certainly follow the physical structure of roots and rhizomes and even pluck them with brute force from the land, but the true nature of these roots and what they really reach for is something of a mystery. These roots connect to something primordial, raw, wild, and complex. They draw power up into our world and express it in colors and aromas, textures and tastes, medicines and magics, fibers and fuel, oxygen and nourishment—all of which fascinate the human to the extent that everything we do is in one way or another wrapped up in the great enigma of the green realm.

In this book we will be exploring the green mystery through the lenses of animism, folk magic, herbal medicine, plant lore, land connections, and rituals aligned to the subtle and not-so-subtle tides of nature. We will meet the plant spirits as they grow where we live and learn to work with them in spiritual ways that create magic and medicine. We will learn to step through the hedge and into the great green realm where we'll find allies for our craft. We will also explore the garden of self and learn more about who we are and how we hold space in the world.

This book is presented as a collection of short essay-like chapters, each building upon the one before it. Some may find the writings affirming and simple; others may find them new and complex. Ultimately this is a book of fertile soil upon which the engaged reader and ritualist can grow their own work. I have tried to offer just enough guidance to inspire and empower without overly influencing your own unique shade of green. If you consider each chapter to be an invitation to contemplation which transforms into an initiation rite, you will be on a well-lit track. At the end of many chapters or embedded within them, you'll find an experience related to what's just been shared. It's all too easy to make our work with the plants theoretical and philosophical when we could be putting our hands directly into the soil. Use these exercises as a way to get out of your head and into the world. The chapters are short and concise and are intended to be unpacked, unfolded, and shaken out by you, dear reader, in your own way with the guidance of the plants that make your sacred grove what it is.

The Green Arte is the name for my particular tradition of magico-medicinal plant spirit work. Over two decades I have been a student of the plants and it has taken me this long to craft anything cohesive enough to share with others in book form. What you'll find here is a deep dig into the way I do things, and the ways I've been taught by my green allies. Plants were our first religion, our original sorcery, and our root mystery tradition. All of the magico-spiritual paths we have access to now are, in one way or another, outcroppings of the ancient tracks. As it stands, the green arte is a fully-functioning plant spirit path on its own, and one that can be woven into existing nature-based spiritualities as well.

None of what is written here should be seen as holy writ or strict dogma. As an American-born person of Irish and British ancestry, I have struggled with a certain type of disconnect from my ancestral ways over my life. Their lore inspires me, their traditions nourish me, but I am still to some degree disconnected. What I share here is rooted in the lore and ways of my ancestors as best I can understand them, but is fully dressed in leafy garlands of personal gnosis, direct experience, and much experimentation. What you find on these pages serves to be worked as a framework for your own verdant arte and craft. Whether you are already engaged in an animist, pagan, nature-based, or craft-based tradition or are completely new to the work, there are plentiful seeds here for you.

I hope you enjoy the journey.

By Oak and Pine and Ivy and Vine,

Josh Williams

THE GREEN ARTE

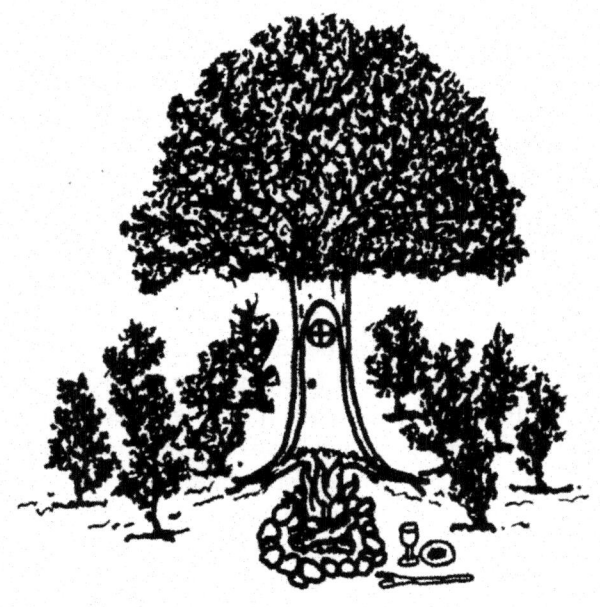

In this book I hope to call you into the primordial forest, that mystical realm that holds the root of our plant spirit work. From there, you will be guided into deep and personal allyships with the mighty green spirits and led into the artes of magic, medicine, ritual, and harmony, and will be called into the sacred grove where the rites of our arte have been performed since time immemorial. The green arte is a path–offering that leads to the heart of the wild green realm. Through flights of spirit, green magic, herbal medicine, following the tides, vegetal rituals, and direct teachings from the verdant ones themselves, we step into harmony with nature and engage with a world of beauty.

Plants have forever been at the core of our spiritual traditions. They show up in our greatest lore, our wildest legends, and our most vivid dreams. There is no more constant a theme in spiritual endeavors from ancient times to the modern day than spirit work, and no work therein more prevalent than that of the plants. When we search for the commonalities and constants that link us to our ancestors, time and time again it comes back to the verdant spirits of the green realm.

The green arte is a living pathworking, which evolves and adapts in the hands of each human person who holds it. The wisdom of this path comes from the plant spirits and evergreen deities themselves, surviving plant lore and heroic legend, and the threads of commonality we see throughout the magico-medicinal ways across many lands—in this case, those of my ancestral lineage. It is by no means part of some unbroken ancient tradition stretching back into the annals of time, but is rather a revivification of plant spirit work whose deep roots have never been severed. The way I experience it, plant spirit work is a green flame that stretches from our first forays into mysticism into the current moment. While the information shared here isn't reconstruction, it is a reconnection to a verdant path that has always been and will always be.

I consider the green arte to be just that, an *arte*, because it requires creative input. It is through study, practice, dedication, and the eventual attainment of skill that this path comes alive and becomes all that it can be. I use the old spelling of "arte" to distinguish it as a spiritual skillset rather than a purely aesthetic one, although both are relevant on this journey. Those who find value in their work with the plant spirits and the myriad beings who inhabit this world and the other will find that their life and their world becomes more magical and more infused with possibility and *fortune*. Profound exploration of the primeval realm of the plant spirits will reveal a boundless space to learn, share, and grow. Through these ventures, we can become providers for our communities, just as wise village folk were in ages past. Traveling on their behalf we can conjure up the magic, medicine, ritual, and harmony to make our world a more beautiful place to be.

No matter how far you travel down this emerald path, you are sure to find great blessings in all of your connections with the plant spirits.

INITIATIONS AND THE MYSTERIES

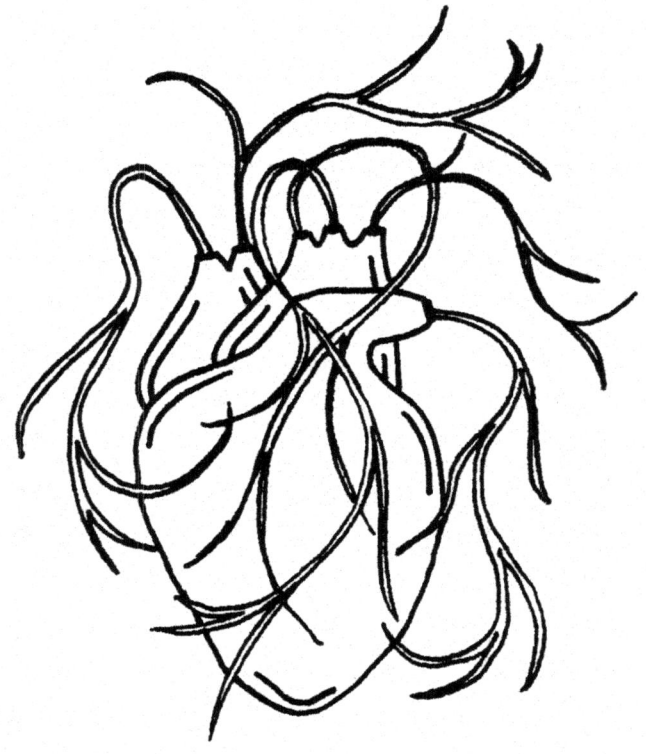

Before we really dig into the mysteries of the green arte, I'd like to give you a bit of perspective on initiation. An initiation is a beginning. When we are gifted an initiation, it is an open door to the next experience. These initiations are endless; there is no such thing as mastery here. As we take each step down the path, we will be given initiations to help us mark the growth we've made and to create space for the next part of the journey. I invite you to be prepared for these sacred markings and to know that after each one comes yet another.

Initiation

Who gives initiation? The plants and the old deities of our ways. They are the only ones who are qualified to initiate people into these ways. As humans, we are walking between two realms—ours and theirs. While humans can certainly initiate other humans into human things, we can't really do the same with the ways of the otherworld. The plants themselves decide when we're ready for more as we learn, work, experience, and understand within their green realm. The same is true for my students of spiritual herbalism. I remind them often that I do not have the authority to make them an herbalist (one who knows the deep secrets of the herbs), only the herbs can do that.

Initiations come to each person in unique ways. They are flashes of lightning that create wisdom and space in the mind, they are personal breakthroughs that allow us to move beyond limitations into new ways of being, and they are depths attained in our work that are so powerful we can feel them with every fiber of our being. Because the green arte is a folk-animist tradition that is, for the most part, one practiced in solitude, the relationship of initiator and initiate happens between the plant spirit allies and the seeker—true sorcery. The old green deities can also offer these gifts, and often do alongside that of the plants.

The mysteries

I like to meditate on the concept of initiation in this way. Imagine driving down a dark road in the middle of the night. The only light is that which comes from your own headlights. At any given moment you can see maybe twenty or thirty feet ahead of you before the light fades into pitch darkness. But that is just a moment in time. As you drive, more and more of the road ahead of you becomes illuminated and you can see that which was only darkness before. Similarly, initiations take us from what we can perceive and understand now and gives us *more room* to grow. They show us that what we thought must be the fullness of things was only a small stretch on the road; one step along an endless journey.

The mysteries are mysteries in part because they are infinite. Our relationships of spirit never dull and can never be mastered. The path is dynamic and evolutionary by nature, and we change as the journey unfolds. Like the trees, we are always growing towards the lights of our arte.

THE NATURE OF THE HEDGEWALKER

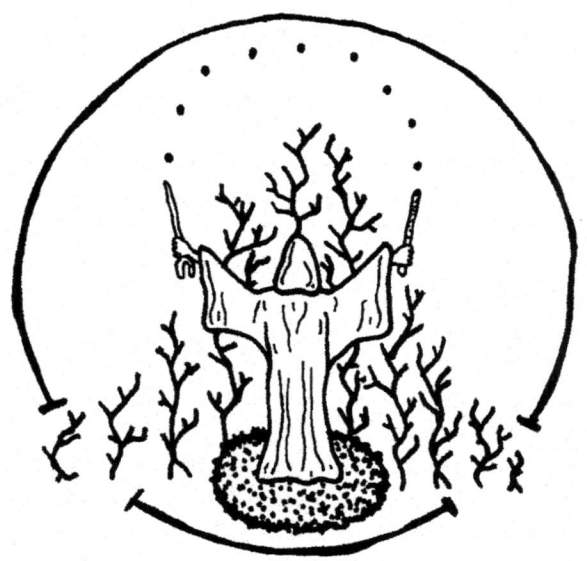

Those who are called to the deep work of the plant spirits are said to reside at the hedge; the boundary that separates one space from another. These hedges, which crisscross the landscape of many rural places, act as living fences that at once demarcate territories and functions while also being vibrant homes to a whole array of wildlife and wild greenery. For those who love these liminal spaces, I say we are hedgewalkers—those who pace the boundaries and cultivate dual-citizenship in the realms of this world and that.

In ages past, most villages or greater communities had a wise person or two who lived at the outskirts of the hustle and bustle of everyday life. They were within reach of the common folk but were just far enough away to keep their mysteries a mystery and require an element of journey for the sincere seeker. By nature, these folk were quite solitary and often preferred the company of their familiar spirits over the noise and complexities of human affairs. That being said, they were deeply aware of the goings on in the village and could perceive patterns from their heightened spiritual perspective.

These folk did not necessarily choose to be in the position they were in, but rather came into the position because they fulfilled a role in their community. It was what they did that defined who they were. Someone could not likely have decided one day to be a wise person, wizard, sorcerer, or priestess—it was happenstance to their own journey. Usually, the wise person who was keeper and guardian of magic and medicine was taught by the one before them, and in turn they would teach their own apprentices. This was done in person, orally, with much sacrifice and effort on the part of the student. Sometimes the wise person would see the potential in a child and create opportunities for them as they grew, sometimes the person would find the calling in themselves and approach the teacher directly. From here, if they were a appropriately matched, the sacred relationship of mentor and prentice would begin and would last many, many years—often until the death of the teacher at which point the student would take their place and continue the artes in service of the community. This has always been, and will always be, the very best way to learn the green ways. Should you have access to such a qualified teacher I will give you this suggestion: make yourself known to them and show up, consistently, in a peaceful and supportive way to their work, until they let you in and give you everything. They will test you, turn you away, ignore you, dissuade you, and frustrate you, but if you persist with sincerity and authenticity, you are sure to win a place at their table.

This work is very challenging and requires a great deal of sacrifice in the form of time, energy, resources, attention, and showing up as your whole and authentic self. Working in harmony with the plants and with nature is for everyone. Being a core provider and spiritual support for a whole community is not.

Being a hedgewalker means that we are fully invested in this world but often feel we are not entirely *of* it. The allyships of plant and mushroom, animal and insect, mountain and pond, set us aside from the usual states of consciousness that pervade our communities and cultures. These experiences can sometimes make it hard for us to relate well with other humans or participate in the same things that others find valuable. We can perceive the culture surrounding us but rarely feel like it represents us well. The simple life we live day-to-day in this world conceals the deeply magical life we live at the boundary.

So, the nature of the hedgewalker is often a solitary one. We can absolutely have intimate connections to our communities, loving relationships, investments in culture, and even working groups that celebrate our green artes, but at the end of the day it is us alone with our allies. As keepers of plant lore and green wisdom, herb magic and herbal medicine, we have inherent duties to our community as part of sacred reciprocity and will often stand alone while we offer these verdant gifts. You may find comfort in this, or find it challenging, but know this—while being solitary you are never actually *alone*. The potential for connection with spirits of the unseen world surrounds us in great abundance. Our 'social life' may be rich beyond measure, just in ways that are imperceptible or misunderstood by the status quo.

RELATIONSHIPS OF RIGHTNESS

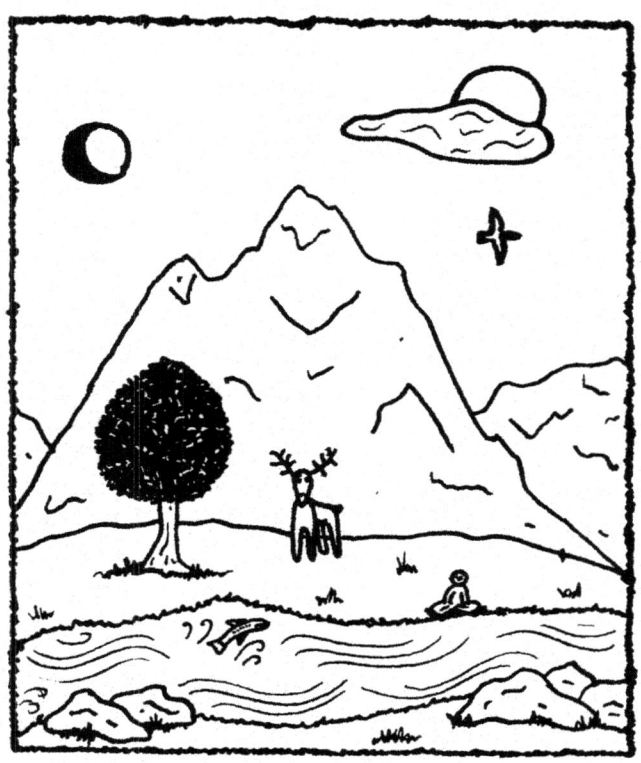

Who are you as a being? What makes you qualify as a *person*? What is it about you and the other humans around you that makes you *people*, and what is it about other fully conscious, sovereign, intelligent, invested living beings around you like dogs, cats, birds, and trees that separates them from the personhood you hold?

Generally, these simple questions lead quickly to the realization that personhood is not a human exclusivity and that we are in fact surrounded by *other people* who are just as person as we are but aren't human like us. This is the beginning of animism.

Animism is a perspective that exists at the root of all the world's ancient, nature-based spiritual traditions. No matter where you look, if you look back far enough, you'll find animists; human people living in, navigating around, and relating with a world that is completely inhabited by persons—most of whom aren't human. This means two things: animism is a spiritual perspective that can help humans to bridge the gaps between cultural differences, and it has a greater empirical testament to power and efficacy as a spiritual tradition than any other on the planet. The implications here are massive.

For those who either walk an animist path because their people live that way, or because they've chosen to return to this ancient way of being, a few things happen. First, we are invited to release the toxic notion of human exceptionalism. We see very clearly, very quickly, that humans are neither special nor superior in relation to any other kind of being. We recognize the conditioning and colonization, mostly from elitist religions, that have created this way of interacting with the world and we see the harm it causes. So, part of our animist work is to heal our own thoughts and actions of these problematic viewpoints.

Second, we walk out into the world every single day and encounter a complex, beautiful, terrifying, and inspiring tapestry of *otherness*. We don't just see humans, we see *people*. We open spiritual senses that allow us to perceive, acknowledge, and radically respect the personhood of all kinds of persons; humans, animals, insects, trees, and plants, the indwelling spirits of land and landmarks, terrestrial and celestial beings, the indwelling spirits of weather and natural phenomena, our ancestors of land and blood and tradition, and even the elder deities themselves. It's a full house, a networking event like you've never experienced before, and a journey which offers no moments of dullness.

Finally, animism is an invitation to join the endless ritual that is a world full of persons. It brings us back into being 'part of' instead of 'dominant over' or 'alienated from'. It reminds us constantly through endless internal and external feedbacks that we are just as much part of the world as any mountain, bear, pine tree, river, or rainstorm. The space we hold is sacred just as the space all other beings hold is sacred. This root-level re-inclusion is transformative in profound and often unexpected ways for the human person that doesn't come from an actively animistic culture- and we can never be the same once our senses have been opened to it.

So, as animists we live in a world populated by human people, non-human people, other-than-human people, and more-than-human people. Now what? What happens when you're in a room full of other humans? You relate. You enter into various types and intensities of relationships whether that be relationships of attraction and closeness, sharing space and air at a respectful distance, or relationships of avoidance and placation. Similarly, this is how we navigate the wild world of people we live in. We cultivate and nourish relationships—these are the source of our wisdom, power, and magic.

These relationships are sacred and require a great deal of work to perceive and strengthen over time. The nourishing element of spiritual relationships has always been and will always be *respect*. You can read about this in every legend, lore, myth, and Faery tale from the Celtic Isles and across the world. When non-human beings and wild spaces aren't acknowledged and respected properly, bad things happen. This isn't new revelation. When we don't respect other humans or the spaces they hold sacred, bad things also happen. We just have to apply what we already know to a larger, more complex, and fully non-human-centered reality.

Respect is a challenging term for many modern minds. We can easily respect the people that can do something for us, have what we want to have, or have done something to deserve our respect first. We often struggle more to give respect for free or without just cause. When I get deep into this subject with students, I often find out what their real concern is being asked to respect human or non-human persons that they have an uncomfortable, traumatic, or even fearful relationship with. Someone afraid of snakes doesn't want to respect snakes. Someone with an abusive family member doesn't want to respect that person. Someone doesn't want to respect the human person they see making choices they don't agree with. This may sound like you, and it sounds like me, too. Here's some good news: respect is a more nuanced idea than we're trained to believe. In fact, respect is quite complex and is the reason why all animist traditions across time and place have concepts of *taboo*, things we cannot and should not do in order to maintain the respect between one person and another.

We can respect another person in many ways. We can listen, serve, receive, acknowledge, support, protect, love, or engage. We can also respect by avoiding, distancing, strengthening boundaries, working around, placating, pacifying, and banishing. You read that right. Staying the hell away from some people is a true form of respect that gives us the exact same spiritual benefit as relationships where we enter into deeper states of intimacy and allyship. Some human people are best avoided or placated for your benefit and for theirs. Similarly, some groups of non-human people, the Fae in many parts of the Celtic world as an example, are best respected by staying out of their way unless special circumstances create an exception. So, there you have it. Relationships of power that don't imply intimacy or even proximity, but all are valuable and add to the overall healthy functioning of self, society, world, and cosmos.

Where all this takes us in this book and in the green arte is into profound relationships of familiarity with the plant people and many other non-human people who share this world with us. Our work is about seeking out, cultivating, nourishing, and working with plant spirits for magic, medicine, ritual, and harmony. It is our relationship to the otherworld and its verdant inhabitants that we draw up our own power, craft, and arte. Carry these ideas with you through the following pages, and out into the world as you live your life. The following exercise will help invoke animism *back* into who you are.

A world full of people

Step outside for a walk. Maybe in your neighborhood, a local park, or a wilder place if you are able. As you pass the threshold of inside to outside, docile to wild, farm to forest, reaffirm throughout the inner landscape of your being that *the world you inhabit is full of people who are wise, powerful, and conscious. They are aware of your presence and are responsive to it.* To help your senses open and attune to the subtleties of varied personhood, I invite you to give a spark or field of light to the center of every living being you can perceive as you go on your walk. Let each human you pass hold a sphere of energy in their heart or head or be surrounded by a field of light. Do the same for every animal and insect you cross paths with. Take the time you need to bring in this practice of creative visualization.

Extend the bridging of your own senses to the reality of others' personhood to the plants. Begin with the largest trees in your field of experience and slowly let the light be present in every shrub, vine, and small plant. Try to really drop in and experience the presence of all these people—feel what it feels like to be in a space that is inhabited by so many types of beings who are truly *other* than you, so much so that no humanity can be found in their type of personhood. Enjoy the tapestry and kaleidoscope of consciousness and power, wisdom and awareness.

You may find the light appearing in a mountain, above a spring, in a pond or stream, or within a white cloud high above. As you look for them and at them, they look back.

In this moment or in moments to come when the practice begins to settle into your blood and bones, by what method will you extend a gift of greeting to these beings? What words or gestures will be placed before them to honor the relationship that has always existed between you and the respect you are now consciously cultivating?

SHROUDED IN GREEN

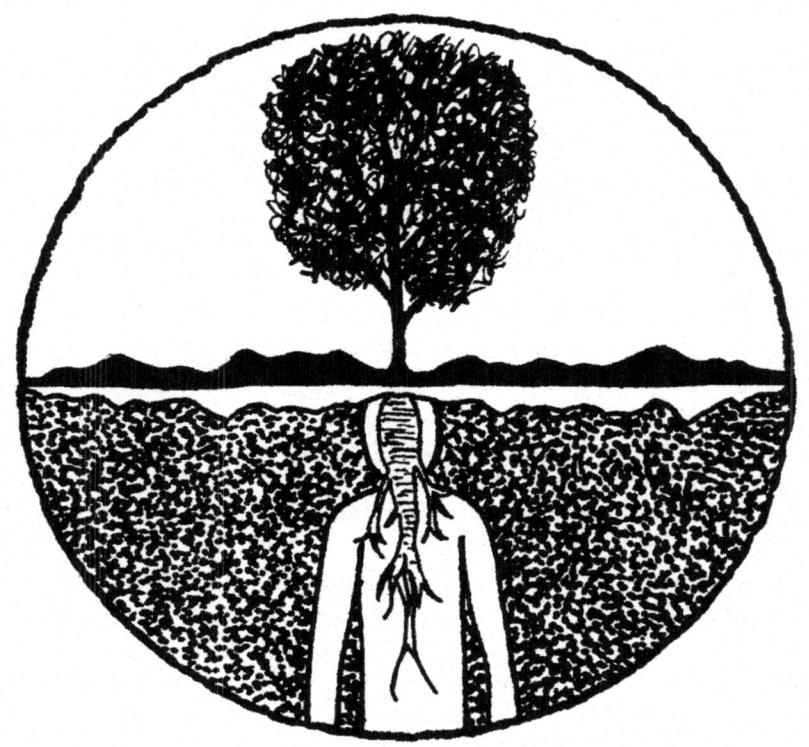

Who are the plant spirits? Earlier we explored how personhood extends far beyond the boundaries of the human being, and how we live in a world populated with all kinds of different beings who are just as much *people* as we are. Our exploration of the plants must be rooted firmly in the reality of their personhood so that we can approach them properly and enter into working relationships with them- but this is just the beginning. The true identity of the plant spirits is a vast, unique, and powerful reality.

The human being is fully invested in this world. We are here in both body and spirit, and to maintain our lives we must interact and relate with all that this world offers. The plants don't work the same way.

They are *partly* here and *partly* in the world of spirit. Where the human is completely of this world, the plant is only partly of this world in their physical form—the part of them we interact with on a day-to-day basis. The trunk and stem, branches and vines, flowers and fruits are an active and crucial part of the functioning of our world, but they make up only one part of the plants' true identity. There is also the root which reaches down into the dark and mysterious depths below. The roots are symbolic of the plants' relationship to the world of spirit, the world *underneath* our own. Not underneath in a literal sense, but underneath in the way that the subconscious mind is underneath the conscious, that gravity is underneath our ability to stay put, that metabolic action is underneath the warmth of our bodies. So, the plants are invested both in our world and in the world of spirit, the green realm. They draw up the primordial, vital energy of the spiritual world and channel it into our own world to make it what it is.

The plants, then, are like bridges or gateways. They connect this world to the *other* world. In much the same way that plants hold soil together and prevent erosion, they also tether our world and maintain it like an island floating in a world of spirit.

What this means for our journey is that when we enter into deep working relationships with the plant spirits, we have direct access to the world of spirit. Through their physical forms we are gifted blessings of the substrate, the matrix of nature. Through their spiritual forms we are granted passage into the realm of otherness. Understanding this we can see why plants have always played such a fundamental role in all works of folk and ritual magic.

But what of plant tribes and clans; what we call *family*, *genus*, and *species*? This can be explained through the medium of herbal medicine. The Chamomile plant that grows in a wild meadow in Greece, the one that grows in your garden, and the one that grows in mine all have the same medicinal and magical virtues. What Chamomile does in my garden they also do in yours. This is because the Chamomile spirit *is one*. This is another of the great mysteries of the plant spirits. Where you and I and every other human being on this planet are fully individual beings—each of us different, unique, and separate from the others in identity, each plant of the same respective grouping shares a single spirit. Every Chamomile in the world is an expression of the one Chamomile spirit. This one plant person reaches from the deep roots of the spirit world into our world in countless individual forms to channel in their unique virtues. In other words, Chamomile is a single individual spirit who can be present in countless places across the planet at the same time.

So, the plant spirits, among many other blessings, act as bridges to both connect our world to the otherworld and to channel power and wisdom between these worlds. They appear where they're needed or invited, by growing in their physical form and by working in allyship with plant spirit workers through medicine, magic, ritual, and relationships.

Living bridges

Find a plant that's rooted in the soil to sit or stand with. Choosing a plant you can safely touch can make this experience much more powerful since humans are tactile beings. Remember all we've discussed in this section. Try to experience the plant before you as a living bridge that connects this world to the hidden world of spirit. Physically connect to the plant and try to perceive the part of them that reaches down into the soil below; hidden from our usual senses. Imagine you are holding the end of a thread that connects you to otherness. Stay relaxed, at ease, and connected to the process through breath. You may experience nothing more than a few moments of contemplation on the true nature of the plant spirits, or you may feel drawn into the power of the spiritual connection with feelings, visions, or inspirations.

BETWEEN THE LINES

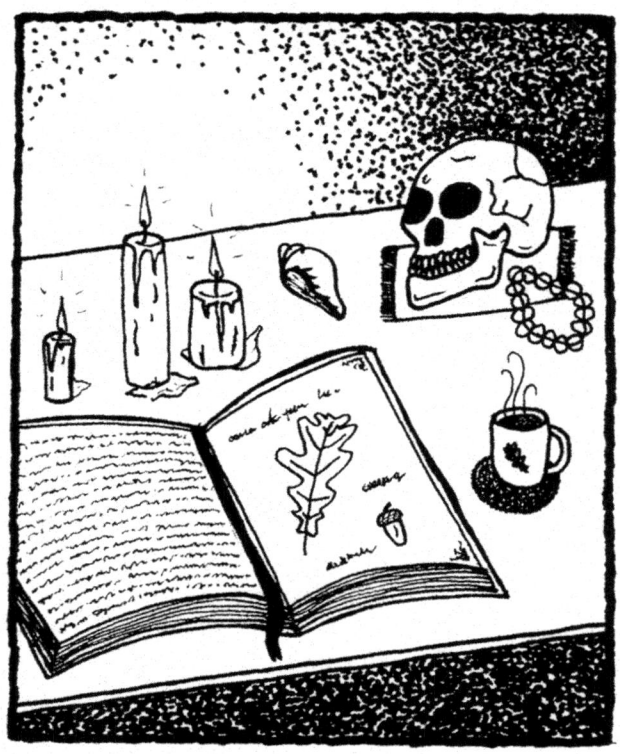

Lore is an important part of our work with the plant spirits. While we can certainly wander out into the wildwood and start our work from scratch, we don't have to—we can lean into the work our ancestors have done and pick up where they left off. Yet, for most people on the planet practicing an herbwise craft, our direct connections to ancestral ways have been either distorted, strained, or completely erased. And so, we rely on the surviving lore to help guide us back to the ancient green tracks our ancestors walked, or at very least give us a place to start and a stream of inspiration along the way.

Lore, also known as myths, Faery tales, legends, and folktales, are the mystery teachings of any group of people handed down from one generation to the next via the powerful medium of story. Wrapped up in an exciting adventure, a hero's quest, or a monstrous tale are lessons about how to walk through this world in right relationship with self and other. Also hidden within lore more often than we usually realize are plant stories that we can invoke into our practice where and when we are.

By reading the lore of your own ancestry, you can begin to develop *spirit vision* and learn to read between the lines to find the hidden teachings held within story. With this vision you might begin to notice how a certain tree plays part in an epic battle, a flower acts as messenger between forlorn lovers, or a hidden grove is the scene for a poetic expression. For those of Northern and Western European ancestry specifically, we can find a great storehouse of plant lore and general magico-medicinal lore hidden in common Faery tales and celebrated bedtime stories.

Part of developing spirit vision is to understand that most of our ancient lore has been altered to suit the agendas of elitist religions. As religious crusaders worked to stomp out the ways of the folk, the stories had to be adjusted to remove pagan, magical, nature-focused, and even medicinal teachings. So, we have extra work to do in cleaning up the tales to extract the power that has been preserved underneath the dogmatic overtones. If you look hard enough, you'll find it!

It's important to note here that lore is not and should not be the only source of our inspiration. Lore represents the past; the ancestral gifts that have survived in one form or another to empower us when and where we are. It is one side of the coin of actually *doing* the work. The other side is what we commonly call *unverified personal gnosis* or *unique personal gnosis*. This means that what you as a unique and individual person experience along the path is valid. Many folks in the hardline reconstructionist movements will scoff at this idea, but from the animistic perspective, and from the general Pagan perspective as well, the brittleness that comes from only doing what's always been done with no room for adaptation is a dangerous path. Your personal *green gnosis* is crucial to working with the plant spirits, the deities, the ancestors, and the spirits of place. After all, what is in the lore was once a new and novel spiritual idea that came in from the world of spirit. There is nothing more special or more valuable about older things than newer—only that they've stood the test of time and have passed the trials of empirical review as they've been handed down from teacher to student, mother to child, one village to another, over the ages. So, unverified or not, what you experience as you do your work is real and has great spiritual value.

Pretty much everything we get through personal gnosis will either be inspired by what's in the lore or supported by it- and these checks are important to ensure that our work remains safe, sane, and consensual. But at the end of the day, to take inspiration from the late Andrew Chumbley, if the spirits respond to the work you do then there is none who can argue the efficacy of your way.

Faery tales

Consider one of your favorite Faery tales, bedtime stories, or epic sagas from ages past. See if you can find it online or via your local library. Read the lore with a watchful eye. Look for mention of plants, anything that looks like a spell or charm, symbolism around animals, or characters that might be concealed gods, ancestral heroes, or archetypes. How can you call this wisdom into your own life and express it where and when you are?

THE CENTER OF THE WORLD

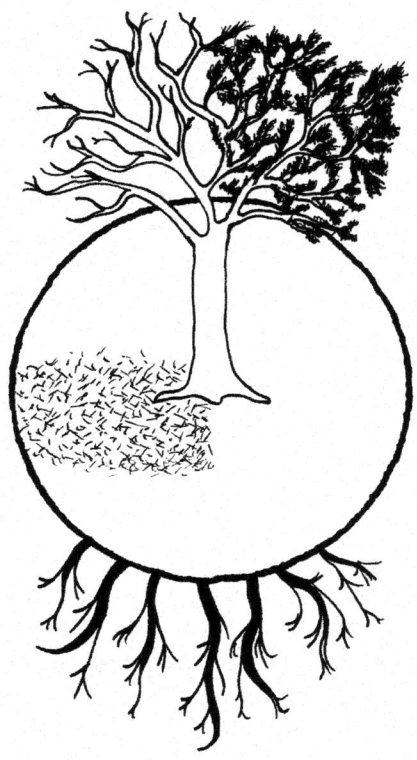

There is one symbol that is so enigmatic amongst animistic and nature-based spiritual traditions across time and place that the mere sight of it evokes a subconscious recognition of something magical and meaningful. That symbol is the tree, and in this chapter, I'd like to journey with you from roots to fruits as we explore the symbolism and ritual of this powerful icon.

From *Yggdrasil*, which holds the nine worlds in Norse cosmology, to the *Ashvattha* of Hinduism, which bears decadent figs and supports the heavens, all the way back to the Assyrian Moon Tree, which has inspired so much of our occult symbolism, the tree appears over and over again as something magical and meaningful. The tree shows us how the cosmos is arranged, how we relate to the beings of this world and the others, how the eternal energy of life flows, and how we can travel between the realms. The tree is a symbol, map, and gateway through which we can access the many mysteries held in the green realm. In the following sections we'll explore the world tree via the roots, trunk, and canopy before stepping back to take the whole tree in as a singular symbol.

The roots

The roots of a living tree reach down into the earth to anchor themselves in substrate and to connect with the nourishment they draw up to grow, repair, reproduce, and thrive. This process shows us how energy, wisdom, and life itself is brought into our world from the world *below*. Where the roots reach, we access the subconscious of the world and the matrix upon which our entire reality is built. The roots of the tree are also the part *unseen* to our usual vision. They connect to and represent the world of spirit, the *otherworld*. Winding down through layers of ancient soil and stone, they touch upon the infinite source of all vital force, which is the substrate our own world rests upon and is nourished by.

I envision the great tree as having four mighty roots which reach out in the four directions. This connects the tree as a working crossroads to the four primordial elements of earth, air, fire, and water as well as to the many other patterns of four we see in nature such as seasons, life cycles, plant cycles, moon phases, and so forth.

As the repository of our dead and that which has been composted, the soil holds crystallized wisdom. The tree taps into this wisdom and draws it up along with the life energy previously held by those people, actions, and ideas that have fulfilled their life cycle and have passed on. The roots symbolize the realm of the mighty dead, many land spirits, and those beings who inhabit the mysteries of life and exemplify how we are fed by those who have walked these paths before us.

The trunk

A space of condensing, organizing, functionality, and form, the trunk gathers that which is drawn up from the otherworld and turns it into the world we live in. The trunk is home to the bark, wood, and sap of the tree—relating to the skin, bones, and blood of the human being. In this place we become fleshy, hold space, and interact directly with our consensus reality. The flow of vital nutrients through the trunk of the tree symbolizes the flow of wisdom, energy, and power into our world and from our world to the other worlds. Many traditions call this place the *middle world*, because we are positioned between the roots and the canopy on a sort of living bridge. The trunk is our area of manifestation, calling in, and relating to what *is*.

The canopy

Much like the roots of the tree, the canopy cannot be fully perceived by our usual senses. We would need a bird's eye view to understand the real structure of what's happening up there and to understand the canopy from its own space. From the trunk, the canopy branches out into pathways of ever smaller twigs. They reach up toward the sky and terminate with leaves, flowers, and fruits. The canopy of the tree symbolizes the greater realm of spirit and mind. It has a perspective, foresight, and influence over our world, holding our reality beneath the watchful shade of the realm above. It's no wonder why many traditions say that the gods and heroes live in the branches of the tree.

In my journeywork, I have found no real difference in the otherworld found below the roots or above the canopy. One reaches up, the other down, but in mystery they reach into the same primordial world of spirit. The energies and expressions of the worlds we imagine *below* and *above* have their differences, but their intrinsic nature is the same.

The flow of life

By watching the life cycle of a tree we can understand the deeper symbolism and power of the world tree and learn many things about our own human experience. As we watch nourishment being drawn up from the world below we understand more about our relationship with the land, the past, and our ancestors. When the tree flowers and attracts pollinators, we learn about relationships of synergy and service and the sacredness of hospitality, reciprocity, and harmony. The fruits of the tree are both the providence of nature and a teacher about the ultimate eternality of spirit: as the fruits fall to the soil and rot back into the earth, somehow we know that it is they who are drawn back up next year to become a new cycle of growth.

At any step in our lives, we can find one or several places on the tree that feel resonant to us and learn more about our journey by contemplating it.

A constant companion on the green journey is this: *what we do at the tree we do at the center of the cosmos.*

Journey

For the one who invests time in contemplation, communion, and exploration of the world tree symbol, it becomes a great gateway to possibilities unexpected. The Old Irish word for Oak is *Duir*, from which we get our modern-day word *door*. In the green arte, spirit travel is an important part of how we do our work, and it is through the tree itself that we are able to step briefly from this world and dance in the other. The tree symbol is an active crossroads through which we can engage with the worlds above, below, and beyond.

Gateway

There is no greater an altar, shrine, or connecting point between us and the non-human beings we work with than the tree; either as symbol or as literal tree living in the soil. Sacred groves, holy trees, and forests of pilgrimage are deeply engrained in our ancestral traditions, and the reason for this is as alive and relevant to our practice as ever. *What we do at the tree we do at the center of the cosmos.* The world tree has always been seen as the middle of it all. Our journeys, meditations, magic, medicine, rituals, and petitions done under the protective canopy of a well-known tree might as well be happening in an ancient circle where the many worlds overlap. From this place, when done properly, we can reach from our world into the worlds of others and seed and nourish relationships with them.

Follow the tree

Find a big, healthy, inviting tree near you that you can comfortably sit with for some time. In this exercise I invite you to simply sit with the tree, breath, observe, and follow. As you gently move into tree speed you will be able to perceive much of what they do. Watch as the tree responds to wind or stillness, how the animals and insects that call the tree home relate there, meditate on the greater yearly cycle of the tree and follow them in your mind's eye from seed to sapling, fruit back to seed again. The wisdom that can be offered in these simple, timeless exercises are beyond explanation—they are truly mysteries.

THE GREEN REALM

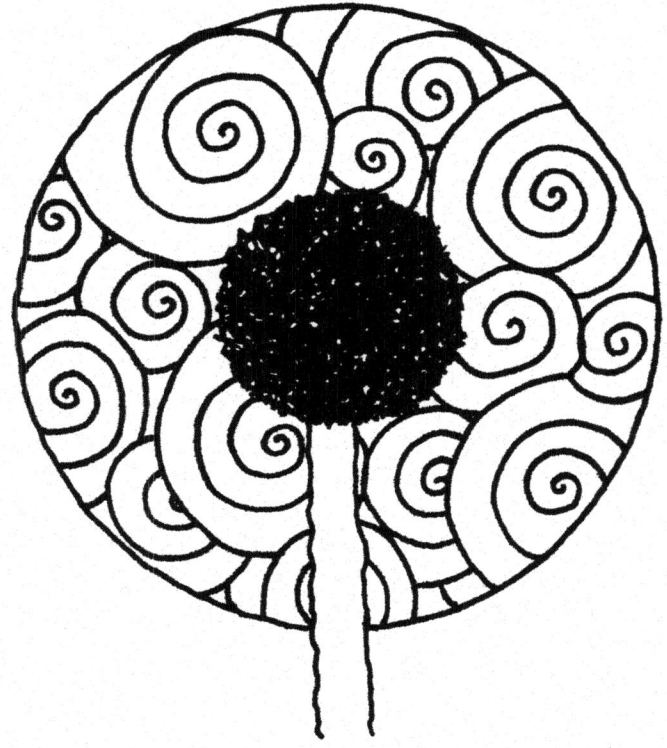

Underneath, behind, and permeating our own world is that of the subtle, mysterious, and energetic. We've called this world of spirit by many names: Fairy, Tír na nÓg, and Annwfn being just a few. Every culture and tradition of the artes across time and space have their own ways of defining, exploring, and relating to *otherness*. The work we do in the green arte is very much rooted in this spirit world, and our ability to travel there in spirit allows us to nourish relationships and receive wisdom directly from our allies without the need to rely on the experiences or formulas of others.

The green realm is likened to the metabolism which is behind the heat and transformative power of the body, the subconscious mind which is underneath the conscious mind, and gravity which quietly holds all things in their place. It is the substrate or matrix upon which our world and many other worlds and realms are built, nourished, and held.

This sacred place is important to use because most of the spiritual allies we seek out reside here, in full or in part. By journeying to the green realm, we are able to commune with the beings who exist within the very fibers of nature, namely the plant spirits. This is the world in which they are rooted, from which they reach up into our world to act as beings of liminality channeling vitality, virtue, and wisdom into our lives. The green realm is also the subtle, spiritual platform where we can encounter the old deities and many of our good and mighty dead.

The green realm is the source of all vital force: *life energy*. From this world of spirit, we draw up life force as a tree draws up water and nutrients. We embody this energy and do with it what we will, then return it to the land of spirit from which it arose, thus completing a sacred cycle of reciprocity. Because this is how life and nature work, it is how our ritual structures work: receiving, embodying, returning. The greatest teaching of the world tree is how important this sacred cycle is, and the tree expresses the process perfectly in all its countless manifestations. In fact, if all we do as folks wandering down these ancient tracks is participate more intentionally in the sacredness of reciprocity with the world of otherness, we will be on a path which leads to great spiritual success.

The work we do in the green realm is powerful. It has an effect there and here, as what we do in the world of spirit reflexes into our own world. When we journey to this place and work with our plant spirit allies or the old deities and forge magics and medicines, we carry them back and find them actualized in the here and now.

As you may have guessed, we enter the green realm via spirit by stepping through the doorway of a tree, most commonly a giant Oak per our ancient traditions, but any large tree that resonates with you and has bioregional relevance for you is a great choice. This gateway tree is conjured up and passed through via our inner visionary faculties in what many traditions call *spirit flight*. We allow part of our spirit to venture out into the green realm while our physical body stays put under the protection of the tree's canopy and a dense hedge of protection. Passing through the oaken doorway, we are transported through a green mist to the green realm. We sit in the center of a clearing that is well-worn; we can feel eons of footprints humming with energy right below our own feet. All of the herbwise folk from the beginningless beginning have a place here. Standing in the middle of this clearing is the world tree itself. Around and at the base of this sacred center, axis mundi, universal spine, we work our green arte. In an upcoming chapter, *Journey by Spirit*, we'll explore in-depth how to work with spirit flight and pass into the green realm.

When working in the green realm, we are in the domain of all the collective plant spirits, their many guardians, the wild deities, the mighty dead, heroes, and many other types of non-human persons including the overspirits of animals and insects and the fungi people. It's important to always remember that we are guests in these spaces and that we are in foreign lands. Our behavior must be gentle, quiet, and non-invasive. We must tread lightly, go only where we're given permission to go, and act with the utmost respect and gratitude along the way.

While the realm feels as though it's all happening in our heads, we are in fact interfacing with the real spirit world through our own inner imaginal language symbols. It is imperative that we behave as such. That being said, have no fear about journeying to this wild green realm. Here you'll find the place where the spiritual roots of all the plant people find their ends, and it is here where we enter into allyship with the plant spirits directly.

Practicing presence

Find a place either outdoors in nature or within your own mind where you can be as surrounded by trees and plants as possible. Allow yourself to quiet down, settle in, and just experience being surrounded by plant spirits. Feel many types of spaces being held, hear many voices, feel many feelings coming from the surrounding forest into the space that surrounds you. Get accustomed to the slow, quiet, non-human ways that plants show up.

CHLOROPHYLL

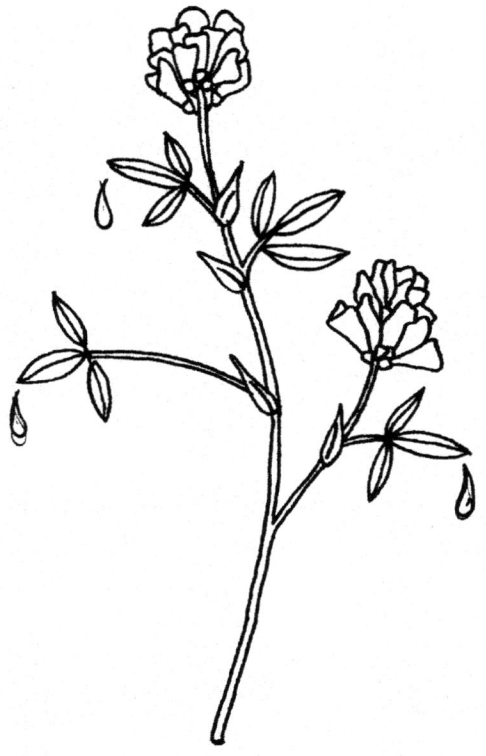

Green is a sacred color in many religious and mystical traditions. From the Sufi's color of paradise to contemporary expressions of eco-Paganism, there's something about the verdant energy of green that calls us in and saturates us with feelings of abundance, nourishment, and wisdom. The green color of our plant allies comes from a pigment called chlorophyll that lives in the chloroplast organelles of the plant structure. Chlorophyll facilitations light absorption from the sun, mostly of the blue and red spectrum, and transform it into energy the plant uses to thrive. In other words, the green pigment chlorophyll harnesses the energy of the sun and transforms it into energy of life; an energy that all plant and animal life benefits from.

It is through the inspirations of chlorophyll that we connect with powerful workings with the plant spirits. First, chlorophyll reflects the green light into our world, which we can work with for magic, healing, and connecting to nature. We learn from chlorophyll that the color green nourishes the heart center (green is opposite red on the color wheel, red being the common color of the heart center), lifts the spirits, clears our energy fields, and attunes us to do plant spirit work. Simply sitting in a lush area of trees and plants and allowing the green color to wash over us, radiating into our skin, and soaking into our eyes is medicine in and of itself. This is all made even more powerful when we do intentional work with the green color which we will explore later on.

We can also eat leafy greens to bring the green blessings into our bodies or take liquid chlorophyll as a type of sacred sacrament to connect us to the deep power of the plants. Chlorophyll can also be used as a magical ink, marking the body for rituals and initiations, or adding to charms and poppets to call in the energy of the green realm as a whole.

Field of green

In our many workings, breathing, walks in the wild, and rituals, we can call in the color green to surround us and saturate us. *Breathing Green*, as we explored earlier, is a powerful way to offer healing energy to the whole being. Over time, our connection with the energy that green represents will bring us into closer connection to the natural world.

We can intentionally surround ourselves in a field of green with the combined forces of breath and visualization. On the inhalation, draw in green energy from the world around you. Imagining it swirling in from plants and trees, soil and stone, land and sky. Hold the breath momentarily to feel the humming, vibrant presence of green. With the gentle exhalation, allow the green to swirl in all directions through your body to saturate every fiber of your being. Repeat this several times until you are well charged with the green energy. You will find that when you carry this amulet of green with you out into the world, the world responds to you in new and more familiar ways.

Green mantle

Hung on the side of my main shrine I keep a large cloth of Lincoln green printed with images of The Green Man. This cloth acts like a ritual robe or cloak, something I wrap up in before meditations, journeys, making offerings, petitions, study, writing, or magical workings. The mantle is a physical representation of the more subtle act of surrounding myself in the energy of greenness, and it's a powerful way to step into a more ritualized headspace.

Any green cloth can be used for this purpose that wraps well around your shoulders or can be hung like a scarf around the neck. To make a ritual gesture of literally wrapping yourself up in green can feel as though you've stepped back into the primordial forest or entered the self-illumined green realm. Over time, the fabric takes on the memories of your many journeys and workings and begins to hum with the power of your arte.

Before use, I suggest crafting a potent herbal tea to soak the cloth in as a way to invest it with the blessings of the plants. Make enough to fully cover your cloth, then allow it to draw in the energies of the plants with the accompaniment of your petitions. Once finished, hang the cloth up to dry naturally. To make your mantle wash, you can work with herbs you are allied to, those that represent meaningful traits to you, or plants that grow around your home or in a space you consider sacred for your work. You can find a protective cloth wash recipe in the grammar at the end of the book.

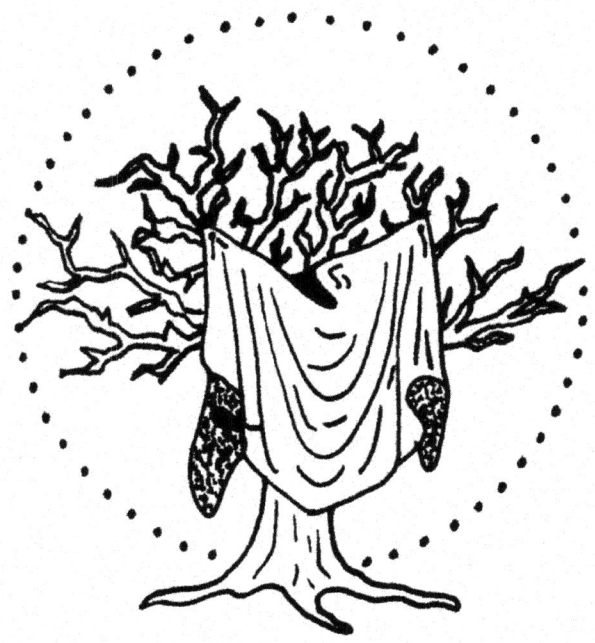

The green mantle

Return to our exploration of *breathing green*. This time, practice with more attention on drawing the power of green into your body and your field, then setting it in with your exhalation. See how it feels to be saturated in this color and the relationships it has with nature. How does it make you feel? What does it change about your mood, posture, or energy level? How does it feel to hold space in nature while shining with green light?

Receiving green

Procure a small bottle of good quality chlorophyll. Explore the feeling of chlorophyll by taking a few drops on the tongue during mediation. Follow the liquid green magic into your own body and see how it feels to have that energy move and circulate within you. As you go further into the work presented in this book, consider bringing a simple chlorophyll ritual into your practice. Mark your heart center with a small drop before rituals, take a few drops before journey or meditation, and keep the medicine close to you as you walk the path.

VERDANT BREATH

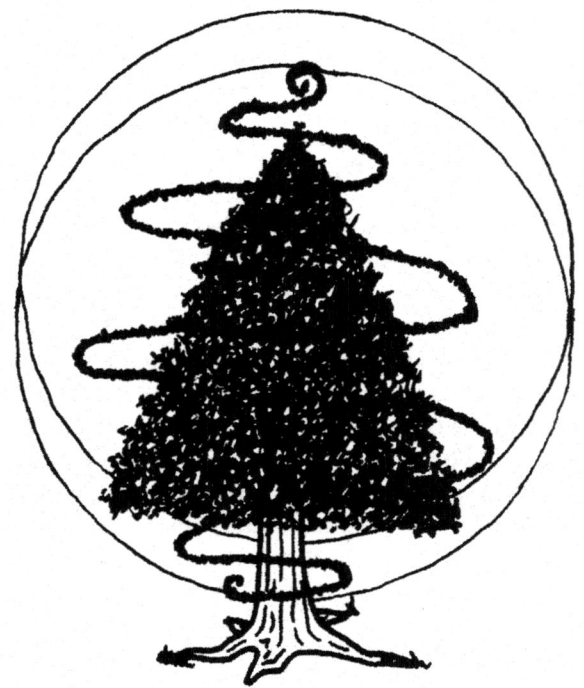

Whether we're aware of it or not, we are in a constant spiritual communion with the plants around us through our breath. While soil-based plants aren't the largest producers of oxygen on the planet (that title goes to oceanic plankton), all plants photosynthesize. In order to do so, most plants have small mouth-like structures on their leaves called *stomata*, which open and close to bring in carbon dioxide, release oxygen, and balance the water content within the plant's cellular structures. Plants also respire (the opposite process to photosynthesis), just like we do. For us, to respire, we *breathe*. While plants are vastly different types of people than we are, this is one thing we have in common—and it's absolutely essential for those of us who are oxygen dependent!

Through the simple act of breathing, we can slow down to tree speed, enter into conscious connection with the plants, follow the movement of plant medicine within our bodies, make offerings to the plant spirits and receive their blessings in return, and drop into altered states of consciousness for ritual and journeying. The breath is a fiercely powerful process in the green arte, and one worth spending much time exploring. Here are a few ways you can start ...

Tree speed

Many of us live in a constantly heightened state of anxiety. We never really come all the way down from one stressful reaction because another follows just behind it. Our sympathetic nervous system becomes taxed and hypervigilant, spun out, and fatigued. The breath is one way we can nudge the sympathetic nervous system, also known as the fight-or-flight system, into the backseat and let our rest-and-digest system, the parasympathetic, take over. While both of these systems are ultimately autonomic, we can work with the breath to influence them quite powerfully. Slow, steady breathing that focuses on ease and expansiveness within the whole torso can help us to quiet the anxious body and mind while also dropping us deeper into relaxed states that mirror the speed of the plants. The closer we can get to tree speed, the easier it is to work with the trees.

Reciprocity

We can use the breath as a simple means to participate in the sacred act of reciprocity with the plant spirits. Simply by sitting with an ally, walking through a forest, relaxing in a park, or standing in an urban backyard we can go deeper into our plant spirit work. In this process, we offer our exhalation, saturated with love and gratitude, to the plant or plants around us, often in the visionary form of red energy. Red is an important color because it relates to our own vital force in the form of blood, and because it's the color that chlorophyll, the green pigment of plants, prefers to absorb from the light spectrum.

This reciprocal breath may be an offering made to a specific ally you're working with, plants in a specified area, or the plant spirits in general. Experience them receiving and bathing in your exhalation, then do the same with what they offer for your inhalation in the visionary form of green energy. In time you'll be able to enter a free-flowing ritual of breath, where the giving and receiving dance with one another seamlessly continues in an effortless cycle.

At times when you feel like you need healing support or guidance from the plants, petition them for their help and enter into conscious breathing with them. As you inhale, try to follow the green breath through your body to see if there are areas where you're stuck, closed off, or in disharmony. Gently lead the breath into those places until they're saturated with the healing power of green.

Ritual breathing

The breath is a fantastic medium by which you can initiate relaxed or even altered states of consciousness for spirit flight and ritual. To do this, find a rhythm that works for you and follow it like a drumbeat. You might choose to inhale four counts, hold four counts, exhale four counts, and hold again, or find another pattern that takes you there. The simple act of conscious and intentional breathing is often more than enough to induce trance, and adding in the visualization of red and green flows will help start the inner visionary faculties and prepare us for whatever journey we're about to take.

The green within

Sitting in intentional, ritual breathing, imagine that you, the real you, the whole you that is radically embracing every aspect of your self is *green*. Bathe in the light of your own greenness. Expand your light to the space around you, condense it, follow it as it illuminates your physical and spiritual bodies. Explore places where the green light may be blocked, dim, or even too intense and use your breath to bring harmony to these places. Spend time, like the trees, sitting or standing firmly in the verdant power of who you are.

VITAL FORCE

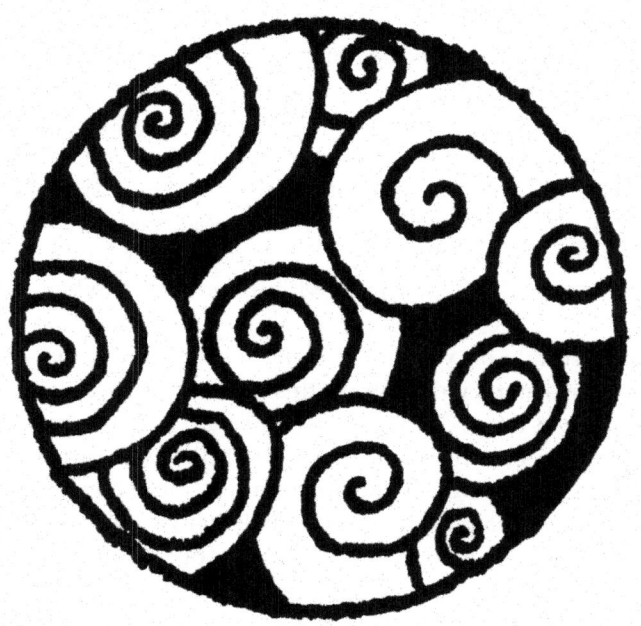

A ll medicine traditions across the ages have an understanding of *vital force*—the essence of life that courses through every living being and through all of nature. This vital force is what we work with in herbal medicine and in our plant spirit magic, and it is one of the great mysteries of the green realm.

Known in various traditions and cultures as qi, chi, prana, mana, pneuma, and spirit, this enigmatic force is the very stuff of life. Vital force is what allows the moving to move, the growing to grow, and the many tides of nature to ebb and flow. Its presence defines what we call *living* and its absence defines what we call *dead*, but in actuality it is ever-present in everything and everyone that exists. It is the thread upon which the beads of the worlds are strung.

Vital force is best described as a river that runs in a smooth, steady, and continuous flow in all directions at once. The fewer obstacles that this energy of life has in its travels, the fewer problems we will encounter. In the human body, vital force is a sign of life, and how it flows defines much of our wellbeing.

Time and time again we see vital force connected to the breath. In ancient Greece, the word *pneuma* implied both vital force as *spirit* and the breath—the invisible power that was present in the living, absent in the dead, and so very connected to the flow of life energy. In classical Chinese medicine, the breath is one source of *qi*, the force which empowers life, the other being that which is inherited from the parents at the time of conception and that which is absorbed from the food we eat. Breath, then, is a direct link to vital force and plays a crucial role in how we can work intentionally with it and heal it when it becomes impeded.

I like to meditate on vital force using the symbol of the world tree. In a harmonious state, we draw up this primordial force from the land that sustains us as a tree draws up nutrients and water from the soil that holds them. The force moves through the fullness of our being, every level, and fills us. As we expend force in life, more comes in—as long as we're well connected and without blockage. We can experience both loss and blockage of vital force for a number of reasons, the most common being prolonged stress, poor diet, polluted air, unchecked emotions such as anger and jealousy, physical injury, spiritual disconnect, and even offenses made to the spirits of place. In a healthy system we expend energy while at the same time drawing in more from the world above and around us—the sun, the moon, the stars, the winds, the air, and especially the plants. The tree does this by gathering light from the sun and carbon dioxide from the air. Vital force, then, is coming in from everywhere and being expressed from everywhere at all times.

Within our physical bodies there are three spaces where this vital force is gathered in a more intentional way. Here, it is condensed and stored to keep us alive, thriving, and stocked up for times when that's needed. I call these three energetic centers *pools*, and they are likened to bowls, cauldrons, or vortexes in which the energy of life is worked. This has been a way of exploring the internal structure of energy systems within the body that I have found to be incredibly helpful and direct, and one which is hinted at in many traditions from across the Celtic lands.

The crown

The crown pool is located in the lower part of the body, from the solar plexus region to the soles of the feet. It is likened to the crown of a tree that rests on top of the soil and reaches down into the earth below through the roots. This pool gathers heavy, cool, dense energy, which is sustaining to the physical form and can be completely still. Our flesh, muscle, bone, connective tissues, and energy levels are influenced by this pool, as are the physical areas under its direct influence, such as the lower back, organs of digestion and elimination, sexual organs, legs, and feet. This pool connects to the elements of earth and water, aligning to roots that plunge into the earth and draw up water.

The heart

At the center of our being, aligned to the thoracic cavity of heart and lungs, is the heart pool. This reserve, the trunk of the tree, gathers energy from below, above, and all around. It is primarily concerned with the collection of incoming information, which is first interpreted by the heart, then by the other thinking organs of gut and brain. The heart pool is fluid, warm, and sometimes fiery. It flows in the shape of a torus. This energy center relates to the health of our hearts and lungs, which are the spaces where we communicate with the world of spirit and the subtle languages of our own world. The heart pool extends down the arms and into the hands, allowing us to infuse the central energy of our beings into the magic and medicine we craft. It also makes our touch powerful and allows us to communicate more directly with plant allies and spirits of place. This pool is connected to the element of fire.

The canopy

This pool resides in the head and is aligned to brain, eyes, mouth, voice, neck, hearing, and the central and peripheral nervous systems. The canopy pool draws in energy from the atmosphere, the sun, stars, and moon, and our breath. This area rules thinking, breathing, speaking, communicating, the nervous system, and inspiration. It is light, dry, in constant motion, and is connected to the element air.

When the pools are full and flowing in the ways that are appropriate to them, we experience states of health, harmony, and power. Through them we're connected to the great tides of nature's energy from within our own bodies. When we're unable to gather enough vital force from the world around us, or when it can't flow easily to each pool and thus each part of our being, the pools can become low or even dried up causing issues of deficiency, lack, weakness, and disconnect in the related areas. Sometimes we take on too much vital force or hoard it within ourselves, often as a result of fear, scarcity, or self-protective measures, which can cause too much energy in the pools leading to hyperactive functioning, buildup, backup, overactive responses from body systems, spinning out, overflowing of emotions like anger and resentment, and eventually burnout. Energy must be able to flow in, move easily through the whole being, fill what is empty, drain what is overflowing, and nourish every part of our beings. Visualizing the movement of vital force in the body in this way can help us to explore our own disharmonies and create healing where and when it's needed.

The flow of vital force through our bodies is one of the ways we are directly connected to nature and one of the ways we actively participate in nature. One thing that will always link us to the wholeness of life is this vital force—everything that is remains part of the flow. When we are like a strong tree, a healthy river, a well-filled cup, we are best able to do our duties in the places where we have influence and responsibility. The flow of vital force is also crucial in many of our workings in the arte. Magic is easier, medicine making is more powerful, meditation is more effective, spirit flights are more energized, and we are able to craft from being *part of* rather than by forcing things with just our own energy and resources. The greater your relationship with vitality is and the better it moves through you, the better your arte and personal wellness.

So, how do we work with vital force? Here are a few simple techniques I invite you to explore.

Breathing

As we explored in the previous chapter, breath is a crucial part of our work. The breath is deeply connected to the gathering of vital force and its flow through the body, so while we're learning to *breathe green*, we can also develop our energy work along the way.

Here is a simple exercise that can help you both check in on the flow of energy within and do gentle healing work where it's needed.

Simply follow the breath through your whole body using your senses and your visionary faculties.

- Sit or lie down comfortably. Make sure to take time here so that your body doesn't have to speak up from discomfort while you're doing the work. If you feel any areas of restriction, hardness, or pain, adjust your clothing and position until it feels better.
- Breathing in through your nose and out through gently opened lips, let your breath move at whatever pace and depth it does. We are trying to see things as they are, not influence them just yet. Simply observe. Follow your breath as it draws in through your nostrils and down into your body. Imagine the breath going everywhere within you, filling you up from head to soles.
- As you follow the breath, you may notice areas of your body that feel tight, uncomfortable, restricted, or completely cut off. These areas are not filling with the vitality of the inhalation and the more you focus on them the more you may find them to be dark, heavy, and even painful via your inner vision. These are areas that need healing. If you're having a hard time pulling this all together, imagine that your whole body is a balloon. Explore the parts where the balloon fills easily and peacefully, and areas where the rubber might feel brittle, frozen, stuck together, or unreachable.
- As you work with this technique over time, you'll come to experience ways in which vital force moves in your own body. It gets easier with practice, but it does require practice!
- A helpful method to imagine breathing into specific parts of your body, one at a time, part by part. Begin by breathing into your head, then neck, left arm then right arm, and so on until you've given attention to every part of your being. This way you can really tune in and identify where there may be areas that need work.
- For those spaces where the breath and thus the vital force is restricted, the breath is both the diagnostic tool and the healing tool. Finding one place to focus on at a time, you can use your breath to gently ease into those stuck spaces. Never force. Follow the teachings of water and slowly gain access by gentle, consistent presence via the breath. Some areas may open up and regulate relatively easily with just a few intentional breaths drawn into them. Others may require many sessions of work to see even small results. Both are correct. As you do this work you may also find that things come up for you in the

process and in times outside of practice. Emotions, patterns, beliefs, and toxicities can slowly trickle up to be resolved as part of our green breath work. This is a fantastic time to call in the power of the plants with the support of a qualified herbalist to help heal the blockages from another supportive angle.
- To call in a more visionary approach, try experiencing the breath that comes in as a vibrant, powerful green. Full of life, vitality, and energy, this green light is capable of healing all ills.
- It may be that deeper work is needed to resolve blockages. I like to begin with this technique and move to the others below if needed.
- This makes for a great weekly check-in and tune-up practice. Do it often, especially at first as you're working through any established issues in the flow.

Touch

Therapeutic, intentional touch is a powerful way to help relieve issues with vital flow in the body. Building on the breathwork exercise above, we can add in touch to help soften tissues, move blood and lymph, circulate energy, and bring more healing awareness to specific spaces.

- Place a palm gently over a spot where stagnation or blockage is experienced while continuing to breathe into that space. See if the combination of physical touch and movement of energy via the breath is more helpful.
- Light tapping, stroking, pulsing, or pushing can be used when it makes sense intuitively to help clear out blocks. Continue breathing into the space while gently tapping or massaging the area to see if that allows the breath to get in further.
- The palms can be rubbed together briskly to generate heat, then placed over stuck, cold, stagnant, or disconnected areas to encourage flow.
- Fresh cuttings of medicinal allies can be placed on the body or stroked over stuck areas to help clear and heal issues in conjunction with breathwork.
- Herbal salves, balms, washes, and tinctures can be applied topically to the areas when safe and appropriate to call in the virtues of specific plant allies.

- Appropriate herbs can be smoldered so that their smoke can be used to wash the afflicted area and carry away disharmony.

Vision

The faculties of the inner vision, that of *creative visualization*, can be incredible medicine in this work. When you encounter blockages in the flow, invite yourself to go within and take a look.

- Ask yourself: what color does this blockage appear to be? What shape is it? What kind of space does it hold? Is it heavy or light? How is its texture?
- See if you can use your inner vision to call up an image in your mind's eye of what the blockage looks like in imaginal space.
- From here, you can get creative. Based on what the blockage appears as, what would you need to do to reconcile it? If it's hard, could you imagine bathing it in river water to soften it? If it's heavy, can you imagine chipping away at it a bit each day until it's gone? If it's blue, what color could you call in to transform it?
- Are there any healing symbols, colors, or even sounds you can project with your mind's eye to the blocked area?

You can also use your powers of inner vision to journey within yourself and travel from head to heels. Allow the imagery and feelings to arise however they do and let them be symbols for what's happening within. By journeying in this way, you can get a more visual hit on what may be happening in your body. Areas may appear flushed with red, frozen in cool blue, blocked by rough walls, or weighed down with metallic spheres. Whatever comes up for you is meaningful in your own internal language. With this feedback in mind, you can decide what types of imaginal solutions you can conjure up to help solve the problem.

I also like to use a more visual approach when exploring the states of my three pools. Allow them to come into your mind's eye, one at a time, and see how they're functioning. Are they bright and clear, or muddy and stagnant? Dark and heavy or effervescent and lively? Spinning or still, clockwise or counterclockwise? Consider what you see, how it feels, and what it means for you as an individual.

The plants

Our green allies are of course incredibly helpful in this work. In my practice of spiritual herbalism, I often say 'treat what you see'. This is radical trusting of the body's wisdom, and it means that what we are shown by symptoms tells us what's the most important thing to be focusing on. Similarly, as things come up for you in your internal journeys and your daily experiences of body communication, the herbs can be called in to help.

As we establish close working relationships with the plant allies later, those specific plants can be invoked to help us heal and resolve issues within. We can also work with a qualified herbalist to identify plants or formulas that might speak to the areas, feelings, or experiences we're struggling to free so that while we're doing internal breath work, we're also supporting the same healing with herbal medicine.

As mentioned earlier, the vital force that flows through us connects us to the vital force that flows through the plants and through all of nature. It is something of *sameness* that helps us relate to non-human persons. This work is simple on the outside but incredibly powerful within. By ensuring that vital force is able to flow peacefully, easily, and unrestricted through us, we can work our artes with greater efficacy and live lives with more wellness and joy.

ENTERING THE GREEN

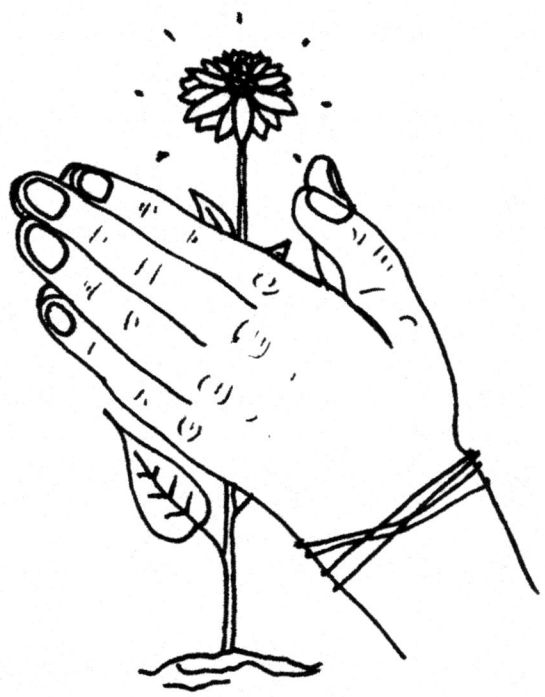

Our entire journey hinges on two things: plants are people and are thus capable of conscious communication, and our ability to engage in conscious communication with them. Plant spirit communication is perhaps the most important arte and skill to tonify, because with it we are able to learn our craft directly from the plant spirits themselves! We are no longer shackled to recipes that might be irrelevant for our bioregion or need, or rituals written by someone else for a relationship that differs from the one we're cultivating. Plant spirit communication is really where the seed hits the soil. It's where the deeper sorcerous work of seeking out, cultivating, and nourishing relationships with the plant people begins; it's a skill we return to every day, every ritual, every crafting, over and over again. The good news is that it's relatively simple, everyone can learn to do it if they are willing to offer up the sacrifice of practice, and once it starts it becomes stronger and more refined over time.

Reader, be forewarned! When you open up the lines of communication, you will learn just how chatty the plant spirits can be.

The place beyond words

Plant spirit communication is unique to our usual forms of sharing information and experiences with other humans. With humans, we use language, either verbal or otherwise, that translates to specific meaning. I can either say the word 'cup' or show you a picture of a cup and you will understand immediately that I mean a small vessel capable of holding liquid intended for drinking. A phrase summed up in a single symbol. We learn to attribute meaning to verbal and written symbols intuitively as we grow or when we are immersed in a new verbal or non-verbal language. Our vocabulary is ever-expanding and adapting as we travel through life. This library of associations is stored in the brain; Broca's area in the frontal lobe in particular relies upon the translation and storage of phonological data in order to produce intelligible speech. The language of the plants, however, happens somewhere a bit lower—in the heart center.

The plants communicate with us in an organic language of *feelings*— not limited to any specifically defined terms. They may share their wisdom in physical sensations, emotional influences, memories, phrases or images that arise like projections onto your mind, imbued with a sense of familiarity or simply *knowing*. For this reason, the plants communicate heart-to-heart. Their medium of communication is best received by us through the heart center, as it is sensitive and strong enough to really perceive. My belief is that all incoming information is received by the heart first before the other sensory organs (namely the brain and the gut), the heart then passes refined and condensed information onto those other areas within us. The heart is in constant communication with the world, and with whichever beings we consciously connect to, so the whole process of plant spirit communication is one of simply learning to listen, observe, and trust something that's already happening.

As you practice and have more and more direct experiences with what is shared here, it will be easier to switch from head to heart and open up the flow of dynamic communication with the plant spirits.

All of this happens in unique ways for each of us. What follows are initiations into the experiences so that you can tune in and tone up in your own way for your own work.

Sit down, quiet down

Sometimes the most powerful thing we can do in our spiritual practices is the one thing that seems too simple to be powerful. When we create time and space to go sit with a specific plant that has called to us through attraction, medicine, dreams, or just recurring synchronicities, it's often all we need to open the gates of communication.

Folks wander down hiking trails, sit in parks, and meander through botanical gardens in order to slow down and open the heart up to their surroundings. It's no surprise that so many people find answers and realizations by going out for a walk or sitting under the shade of a tree.

If we have a cursory understanding of how plants communicate, as we do now, and are able to carve out space and time to sit in their presence with intention and a hunger to enter the green, it is sure to happen. We will confront challenges as we learn to trust what we receive and not write it off as nonsense or fantasy. We will be astonished when we glance back at the 'a-ha!' moments that happen under the watchful branches of trees or in stands of leafy herbs. In time we strengthen our ability to quiet and tune in to the frequency that plants connect on, and we learn to discern the green voices from our own even though they are both spoken in our own internal languages.

When we do this work, it's important to breathe. Come back to your practice of breathing green and begin there. In fact, most students I have that learn breathing green methods in person start getting images, phrases, feelings, and inspirations from the plants they share with in that first session, although refining still develops over time. Never underestimate the power of the breath, the sacred space it creates, and the relationships it brings us into. It is the sacred connection point between human people and plant people.

See and be seen

Another technique that works particularly well for more visual folks was touched on in our chapter on animism. This technique invites us to allow the energy, spirit, presence, or virtue of a plant we're connected with to show up through our inner visionary faculties. We *create* an imaginal meeting ground that welcomes the plant spirits to conjure feelings and further visualizations within us.

To explore this technique, sit comfortably in front of a plant you wish to connect with. Do some green breathing to really slow down and settle into tree speed. Within yourself, acknowledge and honor the personhood of this very non-human person you sit before. Try to *feel* them as a fully sovereign and conscious being. Experience them before you in the same way you'd experience another human. Step fully into the presence of otherness and know that as you are working to perceive the plant spirits, they fully perceive you—they are aware of your presence. What does it feel like to be seen by the wholly other?

Next, call up a field or point of light that you place visually via your imaginative faculties around the whole plant or in the center of their form. Let this represent the spirit of the plant and their living presence. From here, follow the flow. See how things feel, what comes up for you, how your visions change and adjust, and what kinds of realizations you receive. If it's more comfortable, you can begin with your eyes open, memorize the scene and the form of the plant, then close your eyes while maintaining the vision within.

Medicine dreams

Every night when we enter into deep, restorative sleep, we step into a world that straddles the one we usually live in and the one the plants live in. We can work with this natural occurrence to communicate with the plants and receive important guidance and information from them along the way.

To help guide your wandering spirit to the foot of your plant allies during dreamtime, all it often takes is a small ritual of intent and incubation before you settle into bed. Try bundling up some of the herb and hanging it above your head, keeping a bowl of strong tea made from the plant on your nightstand, lightly censing your bedroom with incense made from the ally, or taking some tincture of the herb before you sleep. All of this should be done with mindfulness and petition to your own spirit and guardians, the green realm as a whole, and the plant spirit you hope to receive messages from. The focus here is on asking to be given passage into the green realm in your dreamtime journeys and for the plant ally to meet you at the gates. To go even deeper, try falling asleep after using one or several of the above techniques while imagining yourself standing before a mighty oak tree and waiting with calm patience for the door to be open.

Keep a pen and paper close at hand so that if you wake up after a meaningful dream you can jot down important points and fully integrate them in the morning.

Practice with any or all of the methods outlined above and start to strengthen and tone your ability to seek out and perceive the voices of our plant allies. This will lead into more advanced methods that we'll explore in later chapters, that invite us to step out of our usual state of consciousness and our usual realm of being to meet the plants on their own soil.

THE GREEN GRAMMAR

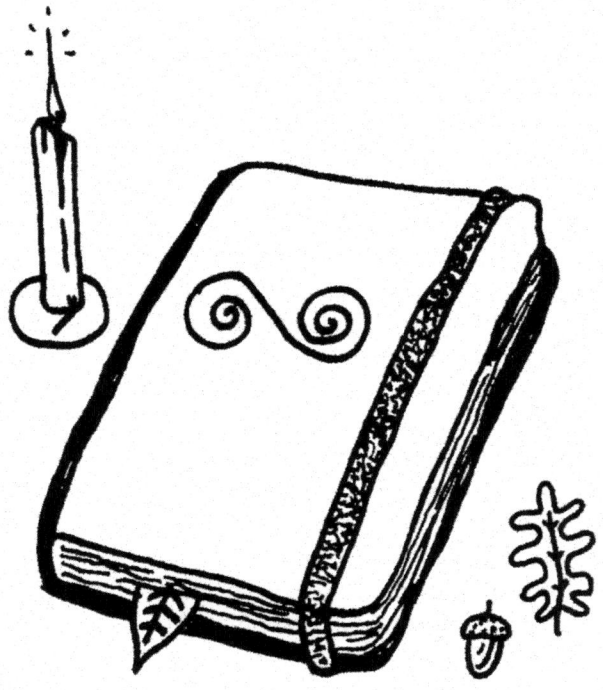

As you wander the ancient tracks of the green arte, you may find yourself encountering a great many moments of realization, ideas, trials and errors, gems found in lore and stories, and inspiration picked up from classes and books. I encourage you, as early in your journey as possible, to dedicate a journal or notebook to this adventure so that you can begin to craft and use your own green grammar.

The grammar, or *grimoire* (coming from the Old French *grammaire* and later used in Latin to define all books related to magical undertakings), is essentially a how-to for your own ways of the green arte. It is an evolving tome that serves as travel journal, recipe book, bibliography, materia medica and magica, ritual guide, and more. Over time, your grammar will grow to encompass the most important parts of your practice and will serve as an effective way to remember what you've done, adjust what needs to be adjusted, and continue to enrich what's working.

In my apothecary, everything gets written down and labeled. As I write new formulas for clients or work on broad spectrum medicines for our community, I keep diligent notes on which herbs I worked with, why, how much, and how they were brought into the medicine. In the moment, I am confident that I'll remember all the details, but two or three weeks later when it comes time to press a new tincture formula or refill a client's protocol, my mind has completely released most of it. Without these notes I wouldn't be able to go back and check my work, see what my thoughts were, adjust as needed, or change anything with any level of confidence. Similarly, our green grammars are a type of spiritual registry that allow us to ensure we're always growing and furthering in our craft.

While many beautiful books exist that can be utilized as a grammar, my favorite has always been the standard three-ring binder. I love these because they allow me to add and remove pages on the fly, rearrange topics effortlessly, and keep a dynamic index on what's inside. At this point I have five full binders just for the artes, and I come back to them time and time again. If you choose a bound book, be aware that pages cannot be easily removed without leaving a blank space, pages cannot be added, and content can't be easily rearranged into categories or topics.

Your green grammar is incredibly personal, private, and powerful. It contains the recipes, rituals, charms, invocations, dreams, and omens that have marked your path and much that has been gifted to you directly by the plant spirits. I think it best to keep this book in a safe, secure place and to make it available to no one but yourself. I don't even open my grammars in the presence of anyone outside the security of my hedge. If I choose to share pages or content with a student, I copy it for them and keep my original in the same safe place.

The green grammar is your way of establishing and giving root to your ways in the green arte, and once the book is open, the words seem to come on their own accord.

KITH AND KIN

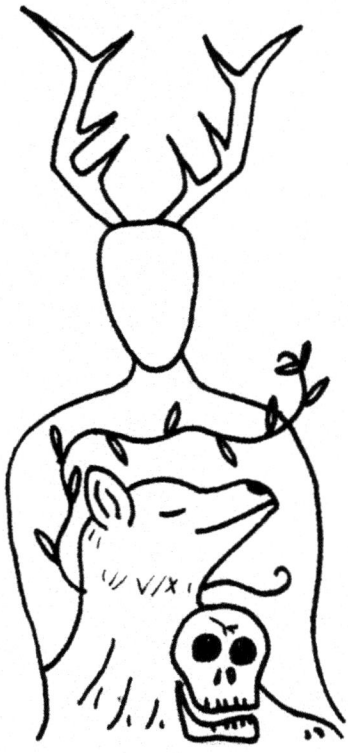

Through the lens of animist cosmology, the universe is an infinite and complex arrangement of relationships. The whole thing from beginningless beginning to non-existent end is a great tapestry that is woven from the ways in which people, places, and things relate to one another. Everything we think and do feeds into this tapestry which is, ultimately, far greater than the sum of all its many participating parts. These relationships are not based on the transactional love taught by elitist religions, nor should they be seen as utilitarian cogs of a cosmic machine. Rather, they are dynamic, alive, organic, fallible, and expansive. They are happening at every moment, in every place, and with every single person who exists. From the tiniest to the largest of creatures, all beings are *part of*.

What does this mean for our work in the green arte and with the plant spirits? It means that we have a great deal more control and power than many of us have been led to believe. What you do actually matters, and when you do it with the fierce magic that accompanies being in harmonious relationships with the many persons who share this world with us, all the better. The plants teach us that the way we journey through this life and through this world has a direct and lasting impact on the whole cosmos. There are no comfortable (and usually incorrectly appropriated) ideas of karma, the threefold law of return, or judgment day here. The individual is solely responsible to be the best version of themselves they can be and to always take actions that nudge the universe ever further into states of profound harmony.

Our personal actions in this world have power, and that power is made exponentially greater by our relationships. When we relate with intention, respect, and accountability to our kith and kin of this world and the other, we step into alignment with the whole of the universe. We get into rhythm with nature and all the beings who call nature home. We begin to swim with the current instead of against it.

Over the next few chapters, we'll be looking at some of the kith and kin who are invested in our lives each and every day: the eldest deities, the spirits of nature, and our ancestors. We'll learn about who they are, how they tend to interact with us human folk, and how we can better acknowledge and participate in their presence.

Check your connections

How do the relationships in your life actually create the life you live? What relationships seem the most powerful to you, and which seem the weakest? How do you relate to places and things, to humans and to non-human beings? Are there ways that these relationships could be nourished in different ways to bring more harmony into your life?

DEITIES OF THE GREEN REALM

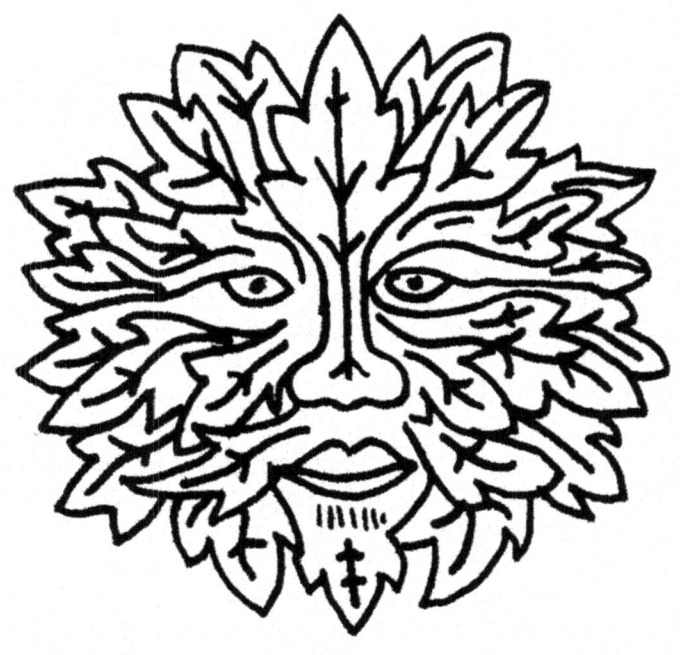

The old deities of the arte are ancient, powerful, and wise. They are not the creators of the universe in the sense that most religions teach, rather they are active and integral participants in the eternal cosmos. Some have come into being as they are, others became as they are after many countless journeys in many countless forms. Because animism, folk magic, and plant spirit work are all relationship-based paths, we are more concerned with how we relate to these beings than where they came from or how they attained their status. They may share this information with us as part of our devotional journeys with them, or they may not. What matters is that they have a perspective and a storehouse of power and wisdom that we can align to as we work our arte.

Another aspect to the old ones is that they do not live 'out there' somewhere. They are neither in a far-off heaven or a realm so distant that they cannot be approached. They are *our deities* because they are close by, always within earshot. The great spirits of animist, pagan, and craft folk are imminent; they haunt the same lands we walk while having access to the many realms and layers of reality that aren't always available to us. They are gods because of these abilities, and they are with us.

Because animism and the arte are fundamentally polytheistic in nature as part of embracing a world and thus a cosmos inhabited by a vast variety of people, the list of beings that one might consider to be a deity is quite extensive. Every culture and tradition from the animist world have their pantheons, hierarchies, families, and rosters of great spirits considered to be aligned to godhood. The folk who are part of those traditions will either be born into a family with a patron deity whom they will dedicate themselves to, find or be found by a deity as part of initiatory rituals, or link up with a deity due to shared interests or continued crossing of paths. It is common in animist traditions that each human has one or several patron deities that they turn to for teaching, guidance, protection, and companionship. These are truly relationships of power and often form the bridge that connects one to the realm of the great ones.

In the green arte, folks tend to focus on deities who have an affinity with vegetation, agriculture, herbalism, land protection, or the plant spirits themselves. These deities are already aligned to the work we're interested in, are usually the ones who call us, and they make for helpful allies in our personal development. As you journey down the verdant tracks of the herbwise, you're encouraged to explore the lore of your own ancestry to learn more about the great spirits they count among their pantheon. Study of the lore is a great way to have your attention grabbed by a deity who stands out so that you can get to know them better through further research, journeywork, and devotions.

The great green god

Hidden amongst the old ones of craft we can find ancient traces of a deity who is very much alive and invested in the narrative of our world. He goes by many names, and has become the patron of the green arte and of many folks who walk a green path of magic and medicine. He is the vegetation face of the old horned god of nature and has special interest in the plant spirits and in the places where the plants grow.

The Great Green God, also known as The Green Man, has reflexes in all of our shared ancestral cultures. Osiris, Attis, Enkidu, Dionysus, Bacchus, Viridios, Jarylo, and Jack are just a few of his names as he appears in diverse cultures and traditions across time and place. The Great Green God is the keeper of the verdant life force, holder of the gates of birth and death, watcher of the boundary between our world and the green realm, special protector of the plant spirits, guardian of the plant mysteries, and charmer of the seasons. He sits in the green realm at the center of the primordial forest where all plants have their spiritual roots. Through his endless life cycle the plants dance their dance of growth, fruiting, harvest, and compost, and he follows along with them from seed to sacrifice as an embodiment of that green mystery. He holds all knowledge concerning the plant spirits and knows all the ways of green magic and medicine.

We connect with The Great Green God to access further depths of the green realm, and to learn the mysteries that make us eligible for more immersive initiations into our plant work. As King of the Forest and Lord of Leaves, it is he who grants permission for us to jump the hedge and become citizens of two worlds. He is also the great spirit who bestows the plant familiar or ally on the seeker. Through his sage guidance we are led in journey and ritual to the plants that he knows are best suited to the work we must do.

The Great Green God often appears as a man covered in foliage sprouting from his own body. Ivy, Vine, Acanthus, Oak, Fern, Fig, Linden, and Pine are all common plants for him to cloak himself in, and each expression brings out a different tone of his complex personality.

You can meet The Great Evergreen God by venturing out into wild sylvan spaces, quieting, and invoking him in your heart. He speaks often through the trees by the rustling of their leaves or the patterns of sunlight they cast on the ground. He can be given offerings of wine, honey, aromatic incense, dark bread, and fruits like figs, apples, berries, and song. He can also be found in walled gardens, city parks, and even around houseplants. Wherever the virtues of the plant spirits and the vital force of life flows you will find him there.

But The Great Green God doesn't exist alone ...

The sovereign goddess of land

Paired with The Great Green God is the Land Goddess whom he protects as her consort, guardian, and child. From her soil-body emerges all plant life; the dark mystery of the ground below likened to a great womb, which is the gateway of life and death guarded by The Green God.

The Land Goddess is the Earth Mother who we find in every nature-based tradition across time and place, but we approach her in a way that removes the limiting responsibilities of cosmic motherhood. Here, she is *our* goddess and can appear to us and connect with us in unlimited ways. She is the indwelling spirit of all land, but especially and most importantly the land we're on right here, right now. Wherever you happen to be in this moment, she is there as the land, and this is her most meaningful face for you as an individual where and when you are. The specific landscapes that make the place you're in a special one are features of her physical form and speak about the face she shows to you.

The Land Goddess is known by many names and in many guises. She is keeper of the earth mysteries, giver of life, receiver of the dead, giver of the flowers, and orchestrator of the subtle rhythms of life. The seasons dance around her as she dances with her Green Lord. As a deity of the plants, she is concerned with healing, medicine, stewardship, soil, fungi, and the roots of things. She is the blossoming of spring, the fertile power of summer, the deep sigh of release in the autumn, and the harsh cold of winter.

The Land Goddess can be encountered wherever you may be. Touching the soles of your bare feet to soil or the bed of a gentle stream will put you into direct contact with her presence if you listen closely enough. The nourishing satiety of food is her sacrament, and gravity is her warm embrace. She can be given offerings of fragrant leaves, honey wine, floral incense, herbal teas crafted from plants grown in your garden, hand-kneaded bread, song, dance, and the energy and love of your protection and stewardship of her sacred body—the land.

The story

One very meaningful and magical way to connect to the old ones of the green arte is by seeking out, honoring, and harmonizing with their great dance. These movements are mysteries that lie behind the changing seasons, the tides of nature, and the life cycles of the plants themselves.

We can explore the dance of the deities through a simple story. Be mindful that this story is handed from me to you, but it will *land* in a unique way where and when you are. The way the story looks in my city may be dramatically different than how it looks where you are. Parts of the story may not be so obvious where you are, while some are impossible to ignore where I am. This story is a framework upon which you can build your own bioregional relationship with the great green spirits as they are.

As you read, contemplate, experience, and return to parts of this story year after year in your own heart and mind, don't be surprised if it changes ever so slightly to become *your* sacred lore.

In the winter we find deep rest in darkness.
The world around us slows down and some parts of it even retreat into the mysterious caverns below the surface of the land. We know they're still there, but they step out of our reach. Winter is the midnight of the year, and so the sovereign lady, land goddess, pulls a blanket of shimmering white snow over herself and settles in for a well-deserved slumber. But she is not alone. Next to her is the lord of leaves, keeper of the gates, great green man. He too is resting, exhausted from a year of growing and peaking, maturing and giving, sacrificing of self for the good of all. They lie together in the hidden places of the underworld—the space that lies just outside our usual field of awareness, in the darkness from which all light emerges, the mystery that fuels all the conscious expressions of who we are. While all appear to be in dreamless sleep, dreams of what's to come are wide awake within. It is the darkness of a full womb and the moment just before poetic inspiration hits. And so, they sleep, elder gods of the dark underworld, holders of death and birth, in haunting silence. The plants also sleep. They sink down into their roots and rest after a year of reaching for the sun and performing their alchemy. Some simply die, shedding their leaves and dropping their fruits—falling back into the land through death, knowing that what they give up now becomes nourishment for the next cycle to come.

In the spring, we wake and open the doors of potential.
Springtime is like the rising of the sun at daybreak—it chases away all inauspiciousness, gently warms the land, and rises up with an initiation of something fresh and new. As the old ones wake from their wintertime slumber, they stir with anticipation. As the sun comes up, they too come up from the underworld, the mysterious abode of the blessed dead, into our world. Their feet touching the ground breaks the spell of frost and calls the plant spirits from their domain. With a gentle symphony, plants emerge through the soil and reach

up, tender and pale, towards the new sun. Minds are full of hope and ideas, dynamic energy to make magic happen here and there. The lady as sovereign is the fertile land which gives birth to all beings; plants and animals, humans and great spirits, all emerging froth from dirt and den, home and heart, as if rising from the cosmic womb. Her guardian and consort, the great green man, holds open the gates that allow pure life force to usher into the world. He walks in ancient forest, grows with old trees and baby saplings, frolics with animals, and warms the blood of the human heart. Like a great conductor his very presence inspires both music and sap to rise up in the world—life springing forth from the invernal, deathly quiet.

In the summer we rise in power and reach to earth and sky.
The wild world, with strength and vibrant energy, embraces the heat of summer and allows the raw power of the sun to move through unseen ancient channels. Plants transform the sun's light into energy—the energy that carries their virtues into our inner worlds as medicine and. The land goddess is hot and lush, witness to the great feats of her children as they grow, blossom, and fruit. She finds her reflection in each flower that hums with the bees and birds, and she is felt as the firm earth who holds all beings in a mother's embrace. The great green god is lord of leaves, inspiring each flower to grow as an offering from his heart to hers. Flowers bloom and fade giving way to colorful fruits that entice the senses and captivate the spirit. In this peak of power is hidden the dark reflection of winter—seeds of sleep within the flesh of ripening fruits. All the spirits of place give their festivals and stay up late into short, warm nights. Animals walk stronger, birds fly higher, and the air is charged with the sacred breath of the green spirits. The plants themselves reach down into the eternal nourishment of the land and up towards the sun; reaching in two directions they are bridges between the worlds.

In the autumn we fall and pass through.
After the long day of the summer, the green god tires from his haunts and settles against old oaks to take rest. The land, having given of herself until dry and sallow, seems to shrink back away from hungry roots as if to catch her breath. The harvest is here, and all that has been birthed and nourished and ripened over the past year has come to a beautiful end. The trees in their seemingly infinite wisdom pull back life force from the leaves of the year, severing the connection from that which cannot be carried into rest. Leaves fall to the land and are pulled through the veil of decay and decomposition by the wisdom of the green man. Fruits drop into grateful mouths or fall to the ground as an

offering to the spirits of place and provide substrate for next year's growth. The trees and plants and animals in these cool, shortening days show the real power of letting go and participating in the initiation we call death. The great green god opens the gates once more, this time to pull life down rather than push it up. Ushering the dead, he guides them into slumber. As lord of the leaves he too falls, releasing his vitality and virtue into the land so that it might compost and build in power before the next spring calls on its magical nourishment. Disembodied and disgorged, he returns to forest floor and brown meadow, lake bottoms and desert chills as the great sacrifice. He closes the gates between this world and the othe, sor that all may settle into the nighttime of winter and find their peaceful rest.

Staying in touch

There are many ways to connect with the old deities and enter into relationship with them. The best way is to go out into nature, invoke them from your heart, and show up for their response in whatever way it may come. Many folks also dedicate altars or shrines to them indoors or in gardens where they can do devotions, enact rituals, make magic and medicine, perform divinations, or just sit and be part of the flow. Altars can be simple or elaborate, and should in some way reflect the work being done in the realm of spirit. You could make your altar to resemble the green realm that appears to you in journey or arrange it in a way that's evocative of that space. When you dedicate an altar to the gods and spirits it's important to make it a hospitable space where they'd want to visit. Later on, we'll look at how to dedicate altars to the plant spirits and much of that guidance can be applied to any deities you may work with, too. You can use literal or symbolic representations of the deities you work with, such as statues or printed images, and keep items sacred to them. Offerings should be made regularly, the space should be kept clean and organized, and time should be spent there each day, even if just a few brief moments, connecting to the spirits who reside there.

The green ones of many lands

Work with the lore of your ancestors to see which deities or heroes they honored who had an affinity for plants, the agricultural cycle, forests and other wild places, herbal magic, or plant medicine. See if you can learn something about the deity in your explorations, and also about the people who honored that deity. What kinds of songs or poems were written about them? Were they given temples or shrines? What offerings are associated with them and why might those sacrifices be meaningful to your ancestors? How can you reach out and greet this deity to see if there's a connection for you?

OF RIVER, MOUNTAIN, MEADOW, AND DESERT

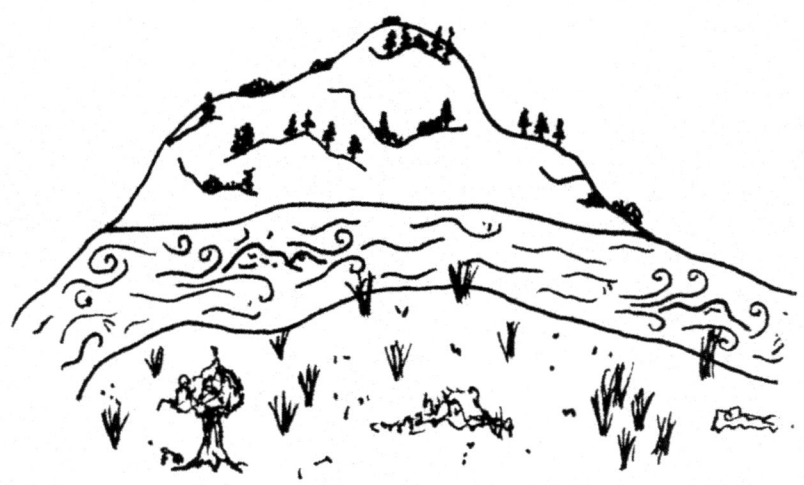

The green arte is, by nature, bioregional. It happens where and when we are. The plants that grow and thrive on the same land that nourishes us will have an inherent affinity with our lifeways, and they are the allies we can connect with in person and steward, which is an important part of this work. Alongside the plants, the land is shared with us by many other non-human people who we can relate to, honor, and celebrate with. While the number of people who populate a space is truly incalculable and incomprehensible, we'll be focusing on three types here: the spirits of place, animal spirits, and the good folk.

The spirits of place

In all wild spaces, and some cultivated areas, a host of beings find their homes. From boulders and rivers to mountains and trees stumps, people of many varieties can be found. This is a relatively complex topic because there really is no way to define where and when a space may be indwelled by a spirit; the seeker must explore on their own to experience presence should it be found there.

The physical landmarks that make up a geographical area can all act as physical forms, houses, or vessels for certain types of spirits. These beings are themselves of a non-physical makeup as far as we understand it but can engrain themselves into forms to accomplish their respective goals or get their needs met. Many of the sacred spaces in animist traditions such as rock formations, mountains, springs, rivers and lakes, patches of land, or other features are honored the way they are because of the spirit or spirits who indwell them. A rock can be a rock, or it can be the earthly abode of a spirit—only experience in the spaces can tell us for sure. This is why we are invited and encouraged to spend time and energy in connecting with the place we live. There are beings here who deserve our attention and who bring a great deal to the path.

Animal spirits

Another commonality amongst animist traditions is the understanding that animals, including insects, are fully sovereign and conscious beings just as we humans are. The respect given to the animal and insect people is essential to living in harmony with the world, and those who put the work in benefit from an endless stream of blessings that include protection, omens, guidance, allyship, special teachings, dream mentorship, and more.

As we've explored, humans are fully here in this world in both body and spirit. Plants are liminal beings who have one part of their spirit in this world and one part in the green realm. Most animals and insects are somewhere in between. In my experience, animals each have an individual and distinct spirit just as humans do which is why they are such unique beings like we are, but they also connect to a ruling spirit of their kind who is the spiritual source of their instinct, cycles, and lifeways. For example, you may have a companion dog. Your dog is unique and special having a personality, behaviors, like and dislikes, coat patterning, and a voice all of their own. Ten other folks may also live with dogs who have equal uniqueness and individuality: but there's no denying a unifying feature amongst them. There is, as we see in all animist traditions, a *dog spirit*. A ruling entity or entities who act as overspirits, monarchs, guides, ancestral leaders, or unifying spirits for all of a kind. Bees do what bees do because they are unified under a ruling *bee spirit*. Just as we can talk about Chamomile medicine, we can also talk about *Elk energy* even though we've never met every single elk. There is something unifying and cohesive about all elk, and it is generally this overseeing spirit that we connect to when we work with animal magic and medicine.

We can connect to the spirit of a kind by approaching one of their kind, by journeying in spirit through the lands they call home, by invoking them in our rituals, or by acting as stewards and protectors of them in our daily lives. Like the plants, animal spirits usher a specific set of virtues into our world just by being who they are that makes the whole world what it is. The ways in which we relate to, respect, and share space with our animal kin are crucial to creating a world of harmony, health, and peace. In my opinion, much of the toxicity that runs rampant here in the United States is rooted in the way we treat animals; no good can come from the abuses that pervade livestock trades.

The good folk

Since time immemorial humans have walked gingerly around both the topic and the person of the *good folk*, also known as the faery. Their sacred places, often stone rings, recesses, natural tree forts, burial mounds, and old tracks, are to be respected with the utmost care- usually in the form of total avoidance. When the good folk are acknowledged and honored appropriately through various culturally-specific rituals, they can be a great blessing to the home, the family, the farm, and the weather. When they are offended or disrespected, they can cause a great deal of harm in very real ways.

Just who the good folk are is speculative and differs wildly between cultures. Some say they are our ancestors that have transitioned into a plane of reality that mirrors our own but doesn't operate by the same laws. Other say they are old gods, great heroes, managing spirits of nature, or even the spirits of the land itself. No matter their hidden identity, it is worth noting this for those who work with the plant spirits: the green arte is radically *fae* in nature. They have always been known to be fierce protectors of both the plant spirits and the places where plants grow wild. When we work with the plants in magico-medicinal ways, we are in effect treading down faery paths and so our behaviors and perspectives need to be kept proper. In my experience, the good folk must be seen as the direct guardians of plants and place and must be approached, supplicated, and rewarded as part of our relationship with the plants we are allied to.

To do this, the garden or cultivated space should have a small stone or stump that is dedicated to the good folk and to the various spirits of place. Organic and eco-affirming offerings should be placed here weekly or on some regular schedule that is kept without fail. I make my offerings on Fridays as is traditional in many parts of Ireland, Scotland, and Britain. When wildcrafting, the guardian spirits of place and the good folk must be honored and given offerings and praise before any plants are approached for harvesting. The seeker should be keenly aware from many repeated visits to the space of where areas feel different, powerful, intimidating, inviting, or even terrifying. This is one reason why a direct and personal relationship with the lands we live on is so important to our wellness. By having relationship to place, we learn the subtle energies of the land, identify where spirits may dwell, come to know the animals who call the space home so that we can respect their lifeways, and experience where the good folk may claim territory. When we enter spaces, especially wild ones, with a watchful eye, and open heart, and actions of respect and honor, we can eventually gain the attention of the good folk and even gain their favor and consent for our work. For those doing delving further into plant work, being on the right side of the good folk and their companions is crucial to successful outcomes and *luck* in general.

Many teachers and authors of modern paganism and in many Celtic lands warn us to be scared of the good folk, to avoid them at all cost, or to work with them in purely apotropaic ways. While I understand this is part of some cultures, I have not experienced them in this way. If we slow down, pay attention, give offerings of honor and gratitude, and act as good citizens of the land, we are sure to perceive the spaces kept aside for the others, respect those spaces, and learn the ways of the land we're on. This is sacred relationship in action, and while the rules of our world and the rules of theirs differ wildly, right relationship is respected on both sides of the hedge.

Observation

Have you ever slowed down enough to really experience what happens in your own backyard or favorite wild space? Do you know which animals move through the area at which times of day and by what path, where the sun falls and shade hits, which insects call the area home, which trees and herbs grow there, and what the soil feels like? Have you ever noticed if the animals have imprinted subtle tracks through the area or if there are places where it would be difficult if not impossible for you to get to? These are all ways to really come to know the land and its inhabitants, to meet the Green God and Land Goddess as they are there, and to really enter into reciprocal relationship with place.

See if you can spend ten, twenty, or more minutes just disappearing into the environment. Sit and let the land hold you, then quiet and slow so much that you feel you match the energy of the place. Be so still that the birds will pay you no mind. Feel how it feels to be here, to be *part of*. To breathe and share breath, to watch and be shown, to hear and sense. What does this small bit of land say to you, and what do you hear?

SACRED CIRCLES

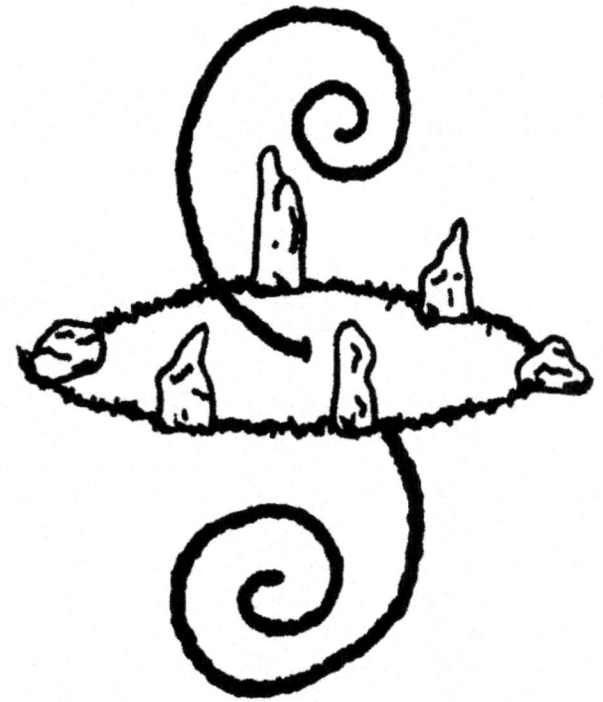

No matter where you are in the world, there are sacred spaces within your reach. Many of us, far removed from our ancestral lands and the places celebrated in legend and lore, feel as though the closest sacred circle is across an ocean or over a mountain. While this is surely true, we're never far from liminal spaces that can be just as sacred as the ones of ancient fame.

What makes a place sacred? The repeated rituals enacted there can build up a charge of spiritual energy. The ways in which space becomes sacred are many, the important consideration is that they exist all around us.

For the seeker of the green arte, sacred space is a thing rare to discover but has endless potential for cultivation. We actively seek out spaces in our waking journeys and our journeys of spirit that call to us; areas where our presence is welcome, our work is empowered, and our kin are eager to connect with us. For some it is a space in the backyard, a tucked away corner in a local park, or a few hours of hiking through a canyon. No matter the locale, the work we put into the relationship with that space is what creates the sanctity. We go there, season after season, year after year, enacting our rituals, making our offerings, crafting our magics, receiving our medicines and before we know it the place sings back to us with songs of acknowledgement and reciprocity. This is even true for the sacred spaces we cultivate in our homes. Altars and shrines, workbenches and working spaces all build up with the charge of arte over time.

So, if you, like me, don't happen to live in a place where there are established sacred areas that are part of your own tradition or culture, this is an invitation to open one up. Petition your allies for guidance in seeking out a good spot and enter into a relationship of giving and receiving over time. Take personal responsibility for the space and keep it clean, protected, and celebrated. Tune into the ways of the beings who live there full-time so that your part-time visits add to the harmony of the place rather than take away from it. Show up, contribute, participate, and fall in love. If you choose to erect permanent markings in some way, ensure that they add to the harmony of the area and contribute to the wellbeing of the people who call it home.

For those of us who are guests on lands that are not ancestral to us, special care must be taken. While we seek out our own sacred connections to the land that nourishes us, we have to be careful not to step on someone else's. Folks living in North America, for example, are likely not far away from areas that are sacred to the indigenous people of that land. To choose one of these spaces as your own is a level of occupation and colonization added to that which has already been done against these people. Those of us not of indigenous ancestry can participate in the sacredness and power of those places by contributing our resources in service of the land and the land's stewards. We can donate money, time, supplies, and signal boosting to efforts being made to protect and preserve the sacred places of indigenous people and work to return those lands to the management and care of the people who have served them since time immemorial. These are legitimate offerings and are potent ways to be in direct relationship with the land without compromising someone else's long-held connection to it. On a similar note, when visiting other countries or places, it's so important to respect the customs of the people who live there. Americans heading to Ireland, for example, should be prepared to follow the example of native Irish land protectors and do as they do. This kind of behavior is noticed by the spirits and will yield deeply powerful blessings.

Step into the circle

Consider the outdoor, wild, or natural places where you spend the most time. Is it in your own backyard or maybe further afoot on mountains or in meadows? How could you relate more deeply to these places so that the sacred areas can emerge for you? Are there places that hold power your mind for the way they make you feel when in their presence? Have you already encountered a place near or far that made it known to you that you were on sacred ground?

As you become more closely connected to specific areas or sacred spaces, consider what could you do to *take the land personally* and step up as steward and guardian. We must step up, take responsibility, and act—we could wait for others to fix, protect, save, clean up, or nourish the land, whilst they could be waiting for us!

IVY IN THE SKULL

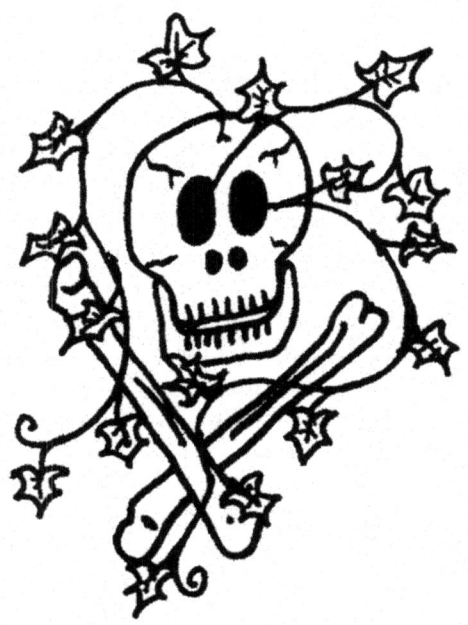

Ancestral veneration has been a keystone of animist and folk practices across time and place, and continues to nourish the magical, medicinal, ritual, and relationship ways of people across the world. For us modern folk, the idea of maintaining an active connection to our dead seems either impossible or vulgar. We have been led to believe that death is either a permanent state of non-existence or a release from the illusory grip of nature and into some heavenly realm far above the trials and tribulations of the human experience. We have also been conditioned to be so disgusted by death that we pay strangers to cleanse and dress the bodies of our deceased family members and even package meat to remove ourselves from the process of animal slaughter as much as possible.

In the green arte tradition, we work with three types of ancestors: those of blood, of land, and of tradition. This delineation allows us to step outside of our literal bloodline and connect with many allies who are willing to guide and teach us. The ancestors of blood are those who are related to us through family lines. They are the ones whose faces can be seen in our faces and who carried our genetic codes to where we embody them now. The ancestors of place are the people, often of no direct relation to us, who have lived on the land we now live on and loved it long before our own existence. For those of us who are guests on the ancestral lands of others, this is our opportunity to acknowledge and reverence the stewards of place. The ancestors of tradition are the teachers, wisdom keepers, storytellers, innovators, medicine growers, and hedgejumpers who have worked to pass on the ways of their craft. They are the grandparent herbalists, the priests and priestesses, the mystics and hermits, the farmers and smiths, the wool spinners and bread bakers. These are the folk of our practice who have turned possibility into tradition through their dedication to the arte. We connect to them through ritual, meditation, offerings, and petitions and work to listen to their voices echoing through our life journeys.

I like to meditate on the dead by way of an ancient symbol associated with the green man. This symbol can be found on many gravestones and tombs, mostly from early modern burials in the British Isles, owing its relationship to death and the dead. The symbol is a skull with greenery, usually Ivy, growing from the eye sockets, mouth, and surrounding areas. It is at once a contemplation of the eternality of spirit and the natural cycle of life-death-life. Ivy, a plant that maintains their greenness and vibrancy throughout the long, cold winter, is an effortless symbol for life. The British folk who were crafters of our most cherished green man faces in church rafters may have placed these symbols on graves to remind visitors that life comes from death, and all life is connected. Our own dead have been transformed by the power of death's initiation and the passage through the soil into the otherworld. They have been wrapped up in garlands of green vine and carried into what lies beyond. They are now our guardians and guides on the other side.

After death, what follows? That is a mystery for the ages, and one that only those who accept the initiation of death can every really know. In my own experiences and teachings from my allies, I have received the following guidance. First, there is no singular place where all humans go nor is there one singular way that we all go. Rather, the nature of our relationships with beings from the other world often dictate how and where we cross over. If we are quite devoted to one of the old gods, for example, it may be that at the time of our death that god will come for us and we will go with them. It may be for some that their own ancestors come for them and take them to the next phase of the journey. Others may even join in with specific plant spirits, areas of land, sacred places, or hosts of animals. We go where our devotions are aimed. This is one reason why individual humans having personal connections with deities, nature spirits, or ancestors on the other side are so crucial to the person's spiritual wellness. Without that relationship we don't know anybody on the other side and may have to find our own way when the path could be lit and warmed for us.

I would like to offer a closing note on burial grounds here, if I may. The places where our shared ancestors are returned to the earth, whether buried or as ashes, immediately become sacred space. As explored in the previous chapter, the places where bridges and gateways to the otherworld are established by one means or another take on the power of sacred ground. When we return our dead to the land, they pass through as if passing through a gateway and, as far as I can tell, maintain some connection to their place of interment. The soil of these places holds the wisdom-energy of our blessed dead, and they often return for generations to visit their own bones. Many others, as noted earlier, become indwelling spirits of the land itself and so harm done to burial grounds is harm done to the bodies of our ancestors. It goes without saying that burial sites of all people are sacred and deserving of complete protection.

Calling the dead

I often say that we need to *feed our dead*. This means literally making regular offerings of nourishing food and drink to them but also that we need to complete the circuit of reciprocity and give back into the cauldron from which we all receive. One of the simplest and most effective ways to open the paths of communication between you and your ancestors is to dedicate a small space in or near your home to them. This space, an ancestral shrine, should be in a position of honor in the home, kept clean, and filled with photos and items that are connected to those you call family on the other side. Please be mindful to only put photos that show the dead—never use photos where anyone living is part of the picture as this confuses the separation between the living and the dead and can cause unwanted effects for those on both sides. The altar can be a place where you recite names, share stories, make offerings to your ancestors both known and unknown, and petition them for help and guidance. A simple candle and water are a good start, but over time you might consider working in the foods and drinks they loved best while they were here, or those that are important to your ancestral culture.

After a short time of working with your mighty dead in this way, prepare to start experiencing them play a louder and more prevalent role in your life. Synchronicities, protection, guidance, dreams, luck, healing, and connections all tend to be signs that our receptivity is allowing them to help us more and more.

GARLAND OF THE YEAR

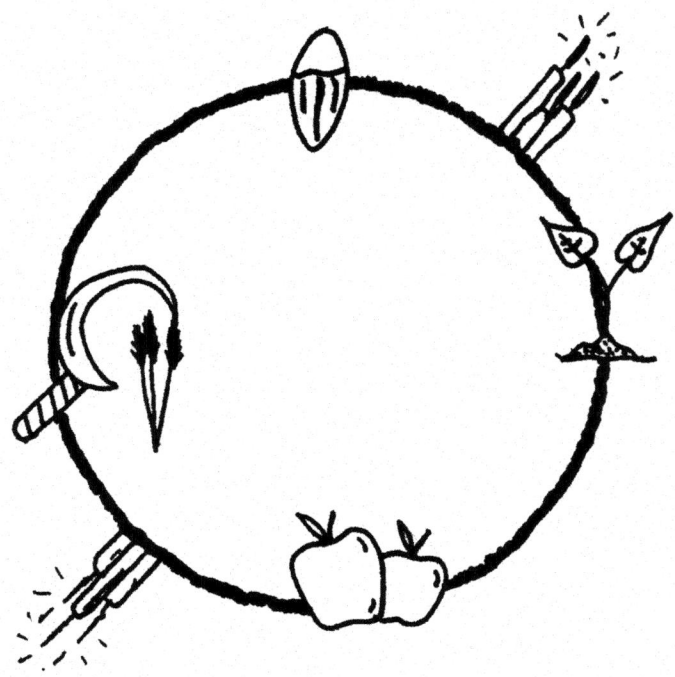

Sacred calendars are a way for us to align to the rhythms of the seasons and participate in what nature is up to as the wheel of the year makes its endless turn. These calendars help us honor the days held sacred by our ancestors, bring us into support of the cultures we're celebrating with, and plan ahead for things like gardening, wellness routines, and rituals. In this chapter I'd like to explore with you ways we can honor the cycles of the seasons while being more attentive and engaged with the land we're on. We'll look at six sacred festivals that appear time and time again in ancient pan-pagan, neopagan, craft, and animist traditions throughout many parts of old Europe, and see how we can adapt them to suit the special expressions of season wherever we may be.

My approach to the sacred calendar is one that centers the wild ways of the plant spirits. Inspiration comes heavily from some of the agricultural festivals and hunter-gatherer cycles of my ancestors, and I've worked to honor their inner meanings while making them adaptable to our current lifeways and my own position in space and time. Ultimately, these ritual cycles are *vegetal* in nature and work for those following tracks from farm to city center. At each step along the cyclical path, we're looking to the plant spirits for a glimpse into the inner workings of nature—and for cues on how we can step into rhythm with this seasonal dance. No matter how you look at it or embody it in your own work, always remember that when in doubt we can turn to the plants for a literal showing of the energy of the season.

The garland represents the cycle of birth, life, death, and what lies hidden between death and birth. By walking the garland and aligning to the energies and teachings of each season, we're given insights into the occult workings of the world around us.

I have come to call the four main markings along the wheel of the year *fêtes*, because I see them as festivals offered to the spirits, the deities, the ancestors, and my own work with them all. These four festivals align to the four seasons: Autumn, Winter, Spring, and Summer. The two other markings which coincide with Summer Solstice and Winter Solstice carry a different mood than the other four and act like the pole around which the other festivals dance.

Below you'll find a bit about each of the six points along the wheel as well as ways you can attune to them in ritual.

The winter fête

The beginning of energetic winter aligns to the traditional Celtic and modern Pagan *Samhuinn* (also spelled Samhain, but I prefer the more Irish rendering). This time marks the beginning of the dark half of the year, the nighttime of the year if you will, and as the ancient Celts started both a new day and a new year with the darkness that precedes the light, we begin our journey here. Samhuinn is experienced as a time when the hedge that separates our world from the *other* is thin and easier to move through. Because of this, there is a marked increase of activity from the spirits and an ease of connecting to them and working with them.

From the Winter Fête until May Day, in most places the days become shorter and the nights become longer, until we reach the Winter Solstice—the longest night of the year. Because I work with just four focal festivals instead of the more common eight neopagan holidays, this is the penultimate harvest festival in my work. While the literal harvesting of food and herbs often begins in September for me, the beginning of Winter culminates as the final harvest and end to the *bringing in*. What hasn't been properly harvested by this time is no longer free for human taking, as we find in lore from the Faery faith.

For the plants, harvest season is a time when their aerial parts are either cut back by farmers and foragers or die back naturally with the drop in temperature and diminishing sunlight. This is truly harvest season, and we see unpicked fruits wither and fall to the ground. The vital force of plants retreats into their roots where it is either stored in rest until the next year's growth, if they're perennial, or released back into the land, if they're annual. This retreating energy holds the same mystery that we humans express at the time of our death—a passing back into the land as a gateway to the otherworld. As many plants are drawing back through the veil at this time, the veil is held open and becomes permeable. The spirits of many realms and many forms can interact with our world much easier, and we often encounter them in much more vivid ways. When the ground begins to frost and freeze, the gateway gently closes as darkness descends and the plants condense in their roots for a replenishing sleep. Hidden within the death and decay of this season is new life, as within each fallen fruit is seed for the year to come.

So, as you may have gleaned, the beginning of Winter is a time to acknowledge, honor, and even participate in death. As many trees release their leaves that will no longer serve them throughout the dark, cold winter, it is a time for us to do as they do and *let go*. Here we take stock of what we've created, nourished, held, and protected. We decide what goes to rest with us over the wintertime and what we need to release to create space for the growth to come.

The Winter Fête is through and through a harvest-end festival, so it is well advised to lay intentional offerings for the spirits who have provided to you over the last year. Of all the times to be generous with those in the green realm, it is now.

Due to the thinning hedge, here we can do deeper and louder work with our ancestors, the land spirits, the plant spirits, and the old deities. Those who ask for special protection from their allied deities during this festival are wise as the gates allow much more through than usual and the intensity of the journey can sometimes be quite exhausting. Great offerings and adorations can be made during the shifting seasons to the dead and to the plant spirits that share their *other* life with us through physical and spiritual nourishment.

We find many cultures and traditions holding special rituals for their ancestors and giving energy back to the land in gratitude for an abundant harvest. In whatever ways you choose to align to the season, know that this is a time to slow down, solidify, and drop into your own center. You may or may not see snow where you live or even feel coldness, but the rest is due, and it is good to take it.

Alignments: seed state, transformation, the otherworld, winter, north, bear, nighttime, dark moon, earth. The Green Man is dressed in Pine and Holly to show us the life hidden within the death of this season, the Lady of the Land wraps up in a blanket of snow.

Celebrating the winter fête

I am a big fan of keeping things simple, meaningful, and heart-felt. Here are a few ritual ideas you might implement in your own aligning to the season …

- Craft a small figure with harvested plant material in the shape of the Great Green God in the spring. Keep him on your shrine or in your garden throughout the year, then at harvest place him in a small burial mound in your own garden to give him rest and transformation after a long year of nourishing the plants in your ward. He is returned to the Land Goddess.
- Offer a special ritual of gratitude, connection, and divination dedicated to your ancestors. Create a seasonal shrine for them, possibly outdoors with a bonfire, and invoke them by name as much as you are able.
- Make offerings to the plant spirits in general with gratitude for the year's harvest. This is a good time to give special thanks to any plant spirits that you have become close to over the year.
- Work charms of warding and protection for your home, business, and land during the dark months. Craft apotropaic door wreaths in a clockwise spiral using evergreens. Bury or burn this charm when the light returns.

- Lay on the bare earth underneath a tree who is shedding their leaves. Work with the tree spirit to let go of whatever it is you need to be freed from. Winter is the nocturnal and rest phase of the year, so consider what you do and do not want to take to bed with you.
- Take stock of all the medicines you've made from this year's harvest and foraging. Bring it all out and offer a few drops of tinctures, small pinches of tea blends, dabs of oxymels, and so forth to the Land Goddess and the spirits of place in gratitude for their many gifts to you.
- Connect with a plant ally that carries light, warmth, and potency for you. Make a small sachet or charm bag with some of this ally and work with them in their root form as you make it through the dark night of the year.
- Gather any charms, amulets, bundles, incense, or anything else you've crafted and no longer need. Go through your dried herb collection and see if any have become spent, sun-bleached, tired, or have lost their aroma or coloring. Return them to the land or place them back with the plant you originally harvested from.
- Decorate altars and shrines with seasonal colors and affects. I like using dried orange slices, pine cones, and pine boughs for this festival.
- Make space for the ancestors and for medicines that help bring on restorative sleep, relaxation of muscles, building of the blood, visionary dreams, and nourishing of the body.
- Put out feeders for birds, squirrels, and other animals who share their space with you.
- Meditate on life within death through the process of decay, compost, seeding, dormancy, and new growth in the spring.

The dark solstice

This Solstice falls on the longest night and shortest day of the year. Aligned with Yule, the Dark Solstice sits halfway between our acknowledgement of death and the energy of birth at the next fête. This is the space between death and birth, the wisdom which can only be known by those who have taken the initiation of passing through.

This is a time to not only acknowledge the mysteries, the many things we don't know, but to actively celebrate the *not-knowingness* of it all. Lean fully into the secrets of nature and find power therein. This is an invitation rarely extended to us in our world of instant gratification and all questions answered, and there is great magic in it. I consider the Dark and Bright Solstices to be *poles* of the yearly cycle and count them as separate from the usual four fêtes.

At the Dark Solstice I like to smolder evergreen allies in my home to cleanse and uplift at this dark, cold time of year. My shrines are decorated with evergreens, warming herbs like cinnamon and clove, images of spirals, and finger labyrinths to trace as I enter into trance.

I celebrate this festival for three days; three *nameless days* that sit outside of usual time and outside of what we usually have access to—the mysteries. The day before the Solstice, the day of, and the day after are each marked with special time dedicated to meditation, prayers, workings, medicine making, and contemplating what cannot be directly contemplated. I keep three candles on my main shrine for this festival and light one each day. Day one is a red candle representing sacrifice and death. Day two, Solstice day, is a black candle representing the mysteries. Day three is a green candle representing life and rebirth. Over the course of the three nameless days we move from death, through the mysteries, into life—entering on one side of the solstice and emerging on the other.

Traditionally, Yule was a time of danger and potential chaos. The Wild Hunt of the old Horned God of countless British tales could pass through on the freezing winds and collect the unfortunate soul who was outside at the wrong time. It is a good idea to stay inside where it's warm and keep candles and hot tea on the ready.

The spring fête

At what aligns to the traditional date of Imbolc, we celebrate the beginning of Spring. This festival is still within the dark half of the year, but signs of the land waking up and the power of the plant spirits moving back into our world are becoming apparent.

From Winter Solstice, the days become longer each day. By Spring's beginning we can really start to experience this and may even begin changing our clothing as the days become less cold. This is the rekindling of the sacred fire and time when goddesses of spring, hearth, and good fortune are often invoked and honored. The fire light casts out the darkness and inauspiciousness, imbuing the atmosphere with hope and growth.

At the Spring Fête I like to contemplate the ways in which the plants and our agricultural deities act as suncatchers—harnessing the raw power of the sun and transforming it into nourishment and beauty for all beings to relish. Look out for the subtle yet powerful shifts in the land and the many creatures who share it with us. The sap in the trees begins to rise toward the warmth of the waxing sun and the magical energy is palpable!

Spring is a time for the seeds of growth to be either sown or gently awakened from their slumber. Growth may be slight and quiet, but it is happening. Often if you go outside at the warmest part of the day and sit next to areas with leaf litter, you'll hear the stirring of insects and sprouting plants. This is a festival of waking, warming, welcoming, and cleansing.

Alignments: sprouting, gestation, fertility, auspiciousness, springtime, east, hawk, sunrise, waxing moon, air. The Green Man wears Vine to show the growing and upward spiraling of life. The Lady of the Land is in a mantle of bright green young leaves and tightly-bound buds.

Celebrating the spring fête

- Tribute the spirits all with an outdoor bonfire complete with poured libations and song as a way to wake up the land and welcome back the warmth.
- Evergreen branches tied with spring-colored ribbons can be dipped in water and used to cleanse and purify spaces and people.
- Start seedlings indoors in pots. As they wake up and stretch toward the sun, do the same! I create a form of the Green Man using small peat pots and start them indoors, caring for this form throughout the whole growing cycle.
- Seeds can also be planted in small peat pots with prayers to the plant spirits for what you'd like to grow and fruit in the seasons ahead.
- Honor one of the goddesses of your tradition that embody springtime, air, new beginnings, or the growth of flora.
- While many traditions wassail the trees at midwinter, I like to do it here. Take some warm tea, cider, or ale around where you live and pour out a warming sip for all of your tree allies—especially those who bear food or medicine for you. Participants can ring bells, sing songs, or make other sounds to drive away the darkness and chase away any stagnant, sleepy energy.

- Decorate your altar with grasses, early-blossoming flowers like Crocus and Forsythia as they arise, and many springtime colors with colorful natural fibers and reusable glass ornamets.
- Celebrate and catch the returning warmth by blessing candles to be used for the rest of the year. I like to arrange bundles of beeswax candles on the thawing earth with all the seeds I'll plant for the year and do workings to charge and wake them.

The summer fête

As Winter is the season of the dark and night, Summer is the season of light and. By this time, the last day of April, most folks will see the land waking up with abundant growth, greenery, and action in the animal world. Also like the Winter Fête, the Summer is a time when the hedge that separates our world from the otherworld is thin and permeable. At Wintertide this thinness is caused by the plant spirits retreating through the gateway of the land into the world of spirit, and at Summertide it is due to their return. They wake and stir from their spirit-slumber in the roots and rhizomes and burst back up into our world in verdant form.

The Summer Fête is a powerful festival date and one that has so many folkloric traditions that a whole book could be dedicated to them. We see celebrations like May Day bonfires, the May pole, and May Day competitive games all across the Celtic lands. We also find specific rituals dedicated to The Green Man in the Morris Dances, Burry Man traditions of Scotland, and May Day parades. No matter which you're inspired by, we can find creative ways to embody their deeper meanings where we are now.

For me, this is a special festival for the Great Green God, the Lord of Leaves, King of the Woods, Guardian of the Plant Spirits. We see his energy emerge at this time and watch as the alchemy of chlorophyll turns the world from snow white or barren gray into a lush green. The flowers will also begin to bloom in many places at this time, and so the Land Goddess manifests as the power of fertility, attraction, and propagation. For those who are captivated by bees, this is our time to keep an ear out for their humming drone amidst the flowering plants.

Alignments: fruiting state, rise and power, summer, south, hart or elk, noon, full moon, fire. The Green Man wears Oak leaves to show the vitality and power of life. The Lady of the Land is bedecked in all the growing flowers which bring fertility.

Celebrating the summer fête

- Build a 'wicker man' frame using fallen twigs and twine. Stuff with offerings of fruit, incense, written charms, baked goods, and douse in alcohol. Burn safely in a bonfire pit as an offering to the old gods and spirits all.
- Dress the tree you most work with using colorful ribbons, bobbles, mirrors, and other décor. Allow the tree to become a stand-in for the world tree and perform your works of magic and medicine here aligned to the season. Remove all dressings from the tree once you're done, and be mindful of attaching them loosely and with delicacy. Leave no trace!
- Visit springs or wells near you. Make offerings to the spirit of the well and the land spirits who dwell there, then collect some of the water for drinking, making tea, and offering on your altar. If you aren't sure about wells and springs near you, find one![1]
- Connect through journey to the magic of sun and chlorophyll. Meditate with the plants on how they receive sunlight and convert it to chemical energy. Participate in this process in your own way.
- Find a tree or stand of plants in a wild space to steward. Take it upon yourself to visit them often and clean up trash, bring water, trim dead branches, and generally care for the plants and the space they inhabit. Even a special tree in a public park works for this.
- Host friends and family at a bonfire and share the last of your winter medicines with them.
- The Summer Fête is a time in my work when we initiate new students and dedicants into the mystery tradition of the green arte. This is a great time to renew your oaths to deities and spirits, re-dedicate yourself to your arte, or start on a new path of connections.

The bright solstice

This Solstice, which holds the longest day and shortest night of the year, stands opposite the Winter Solstice, making a pole, axis, or spine to the endless cycle of our annual festivities. While we honor death-mystery-birth at the dark solstice, we honor the power of sacred relationships and hospitality and interconnectedness at this one. The spirits *all* are

---

[1] Check out this website—www.findaspring.com

given due gratitude now, as we celebrate them at the peak of their power in our world.

Here is a time to give three days of offerings and sacrifices to the kindred three. The day before the Solstice is honored with a green candle (in reverse order to the Winter Solstice), to celebrate life. On Solstice proper, a black candle is offered to acknowledge the mysteries of the spirits of land and plant. On the day after Solstice a red candle honors the mighty dead. These three candles also remind us that the progression from death through mystery to birth is only possible with the progression of birth through mystery to death. Both are expressions of the same furtive laws of life.

Celebrate these three days with a reconciling of just how much you've received at the peak of the growing tide and how much power there is in your many allyships. Each day can be set aside to honor and attune to your allies from the various kindred groups of deities, nature spirits, and ancestors.

The autumn fête

Right about halfway between the Summer Solstice and Autumnal Equinox we find Autumntide, aligning to *Lughnasadh*, the traditional festival honoring the Irish god Lugh. This has always been a time of weddings, community feasting, fairs, competitive games, and initial aspects of the harvest. Many folk, both ancient and modern, also use this as a time to sacrifice the very first edible foods grown in a garden or field to the spirit kin.

Lughnasadh, usually celebrated on August 1st, marks the beginning of the autumn season. Where I live, it's still incredibly hot and summerlike well into September, so I must look deep to see the subtle signs of this shift in the high desert. In many areas of the ancient North and Western European world, this was the last run of good weather before autumn really got serious, and so tensions were relatively high about the success of the crops, and many landowners expected payment from farmers and homesteaders *before* their crops could make them or break them for the year.

The Autumn Fête marks the last push of vital force from the plant world before harvest time. For that reason, I focus on paying my own rent to the land and plant spirits themselves, a sort of pre-harvest thanksgiving. At this time, I feed the spirits of place, the plants I work with, my deities, and my ancestors with seasonal foods, baked bread, honey wine, aromatic incense, hand-dipped local beeswax candles rolled in dried flowers, and the recitation of stories. I place fresh baked bread at the four corners of my yard while circumambulating with taper candles and the ringing of bells. This is really a time to show up and pour your own energy into the land, lending it for that final stretch of growth and ripening. It's easy for us to forget nowadays that the haul of the harvest defined how easy or tough the winter ahead would be, so people took this pretty seriously!

Alignments: harvest, decline and decay, autumn, west, salmon, sunset, waning moon, water. The Green Man wears Ivy, the plant that strangles and spirals. The Lady of the Land is the recipient of sacrifices, cloaked in autumnal colors.

Our plant medicine work during the Autumn season can focus on cleansing the lymphatic system, toning the urinary tract, cleansing the blood, addressing any emotional challenges, and refining our skin care protocols.

Celebrating the autumn fête

- Pay rent! Show some extra love and attention to the plant spirits and other people who share your area with you. This is a time to really nourish and give energy to the land. I also like to make contributions to organizations that are run by and are in direct support of the indigenous people of the land I now call home as a way to honor them, their ancestors, and their timeless relationship with these lands.
- Pace the boundaries of where you live while carrying a taper candle. Stop to connect to every plant, stone, border, fence, gateway, path, and so on as you do. Really use this walk as an opportunity to check in and get in touch.
- Before it gets too cold out, plan a final outdoor event in your yard for family and friends. Try to work some friendly competitive games into the event and focus the meal on local, seasonal foods.
- Make hand-dipped beeswax candles using wax that comes from local beekeepers. You can also invest in molds with interesting shapes that can be used on altars and for offerings for the year to come.
- Using a small tin or jar, put together a plant spirit offering blend that you can keep with you in your pack, bag, or on your altar. Include eco-affirming ingredients that will break down quickly and won't harm

plants, soil, or wildlife. Some options you might consider include dried grains and beans, granules of handmade incense, coffee beans, cacao nibs, dried flowers, small cutouts made from natural fiber paper, seeds, dried fruits, beeswax pastilles, or small bits of wool or felt.

The equinoxes waning and waxing

While I don't celebrate any specific mysteries or observances on the equinoxes, they are times of great power and can be an intense opportunity for works of plant magic and ritual. Many folks see the equinoxes as points of *balance* along the wheel of the year, but I see and experience them more as moments of potential and chaos. The equinox is a time when we step up to a precipice that leads into something vastly different to what we've been doing—cold from hot, dry from damp, bright from dark, and so on. These moments present us with the possibility that things may not go as planned. They're an invitation to actively create more harmony in our work rather than assuming the wheel turns without our intentional participation.

At the equinoxes, take inventory of what's happening in your life and what can be done to bring more harmony and wellness. See how, as we enter new patterns, you can do things in a new way for greater success. You can honor the equinoxes with a few simple words and heartfelt offerings to your allies and move through the hedge with power and grace.

A note on timing

You can offer your seasonal fêtes on the days aligned to traditional Pagan festivals following the solar calendar, or you can call in the cycles of the moon and work with a lunisolar calculation of the dates. Neither of these methods is better or more correct than the other—they are just different ways to approach the sacred cycles.

To work a lunisolar date calculation, I like to find the new moon that falls the smallest number of days away from the traditional calendar date of the festival and celebrate on the following night when the first sliver of light shows up. In this way we're attuning our fêtes to the sun and the moon and are riding the new beginning energy of the new and waxing phases. No matter when the new moon falls, you'll never be more than two weeks off from the standard calendar date of celebration.

LUNAR TIDES

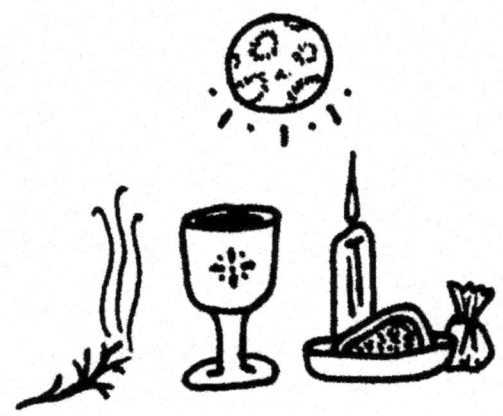

The tides of the monthly moon can be a bit more obvious in their effects than the solar wheel of the year because they happen in shorter cycles that can be easier to explore. They also exert a great deal of influence over the lives of the plants and the types of magical, medicinal, and ritual workings we might be involved in. By aligning to the lunar tides, we can step back into a more pronounced harmony with nature and benefit from greater luck, less obstacles, and more spiritual development before us.

Moon phases

Each of the four phases of the moon relates to one of the plants' growing phases and to the types of workings we are invited to do at that time to align with the moon's subtle ebbs and flows.

The new moon relates to the rest and regeneration phase of plants when the vital force of the green world retreats into the land below. The new moon is thus connected to our deeper spiritual workings and touches on our personal connections to the otherworld. At the new moon I tend to focus my work on quieting down and going within. This is a less a time of ritual action and more a time of internal contemplation and exploration. As the plants condense down into their roots, we can also draw within for a night or two and take stock of our internal bioregion. The new moon is also a quiet in-between time before starting a new dedication with a plant ally, which we'll explore in depth later on. It is the pregnant pause before a new beginning. For those inclined to bring lunar influences into their observances of the seasonal fêtes, consider celebrating on the new moon closest to the fête date.

The waxing moon invites us to participate in the energetic flow of increase, growth, development, and actualization. This phase is linked to the rising sap and sprouting phase of plants and draws on the deeper work done at the new moon to empower the manifestation of new or transformed expressions. The waxing phase gives us an opportunity each month to start fresh, release the old, and call in luck. All works of increase, calling in, invocation, connection, chasing away inauspiciousness, and growth are appropriate now.

The full moon is a potent time of celebration, acknowledgement, and connection. Here the plants reach up and find their height and form. The full moon relates to the peak of power and growth, and represents plants in full bloom or full fruit. Each month's full moon is an opportunity for workings of fulfillment, divination, journeywork, invocations, pacts, and initiations. The plants in our world respond to the pull of the full moon. Their sap rises, their positions adjust, and their vital force is drawn up into their aerial bodies, making this a powerful time to connect with them as they inhabit our world in a more tangible way. When we dedicate a month-long ritual of connection to the plants, which we'll explore later on, it is the full moon that permits depth in our spiritual pursuits.

The waning moon finds each night darker and darker. This relates to the plant phase of harvest when trees release their leaves, and the fruits of the growing season are ripe for picking. During the waning phase we are given an opportunity to let go, cleanse, purify, release, and transform. We can align to this lessening tide to finish up projects, cut off what no longer serves our goals, focus on releasing health issues, and work on deeper intuitive strengthening.

A full moon rite

Under the auspices of the bright moon, we are given a special blessing; a guiding and comforting light in the darkness of night. The full moon's silvery light reveals that which is usually hidden to us; an invitation into the otherworld.

The following full moon rite is a simple yet potent way to connect with and honor the many spirits we ally ourselves to in the green arte. As always, make this your own and allow your guiding spirits to help you along the way.

At its core, the full moon rite is the sharing of a sacred meal. It is a safe way for us human folk to participate in the nourishment of the spirit world while giving the spirits the nourishment of our world. In lore we learn time and time again that one of the great taboos of the otherworld is to *never partake of the food of spirits*. This is because the moment we eat food that nourishes spirit beings, we are pulled into that state and are often never able to return to who we were before—or *when* we were before. This taboo is specific to when we journey into their realm, so in this ritual we are communing with the spirits *in our world* and *from our spaces*. This rite is perfect for those who are new to their work with the green realm and its spirits, those who already have allies in the plant realm, and those who are looking for ways to go deeper into the work. You need absolutely no experience whatsoever to perform this rite successfully and it can, in fact, be a powerful way to announce yourself to the spirits so that new relationships can begin to form. Enacting these kinds of simple, heartfelt rituals is a key to unlock many doors and is sure to shepherd great progress on your spiritual journey.

You can celebrate the full moon near a tree or grove of trees, or indoors with a view of a tree out a window. This rite can be done in the day or night, but tends to be most powerful at the cusp of day and night, at sunset. Here's what you'll need:

- A candle and matches
- Botanical incense (optional)

- Bread or pastry on a wood or ceramic plate. Pre-slice into four small pieces and then an additional piece for yourself and anyone else who is celebrating with you. If you use a knife made of metal, leave this in the kitchen or prep space and do not bring it into the area where the ritual is enacted as metals have traditionally been considered taboo in the presence of the good folk and the plant spirits.
- A drink; whisky, beer, wine, cider, juice, herbal tea, sparkling water, or well water in a cup, goblet, or quaich made from wood, glass, or ceramic.
- If celebrating indoors, you'll want an offering bowl that can hold the bread and drink in full.

This whole rite should have levity and peace. When in doubt, call up the last time you poured drinks or served food to loved ones and try to bring those same sentiments into the ritual space.

Begin the rite by lighting the candle and setting the incense. These are placed as enticing invitations to the spirits and to act as offerings to them.

Now, a simple heartfelt invocation is in line. You can find a poem or recitation from lore or do what I do and make something up on the spot. I enjoy invoking the spirits in this more spontaneous way as it meets me where I am that day and will naturally speak to my mood, goals, what I hope to accomplish, and who I'm feeling most connected to. Call out to the plant spirits of the green realm, the many good spirits of place, the old gods, or any specific deities you work with, call out to your ancestors of blood, land, and tradition. Take time with each invitation and try to really project that welcome out into the world around you. This invocation can be said silently, out loud, in song, or with bells or drums. Try to meet the subtle beings halfway by using your inner visionary faculties to perceive them. The more you can drop in and really experience their presence, the more powerful the rite's effects will be.

> *I invite the old ones of wildwood, ancient tracks, and verdant spaces to join me in this rite. Great Green God and Sovereign Goddess of the Land, I ask you here to share with me.*
>
> *I invite the spirits of place; those beings seen and unseen, named and unnamed, known and unknown, formed and formless, who share this space with me in peace and plenty, to join me in this rite.*

> *I invite my good ancestors three; of blood and land and tradition, those who walked these paths before me, loved these lands before me, and worked these mysteries before me, to join me in this rite.*

We now share in drink and food with the spirits all. This is a powerful moment and one that you can keep simple or dress up however you wish. My monthly offerings are always quite a bit different, and I appreciate how their energies change to suit the seasons, my moods, and the things I'm working on with my allies.

Fill the cup with drink, and address each of the spirit kin one at a time before pouring a bit of the drink out for them either onto the ground at the base of the tree or into an offering bowl, which will be taken outside and emptied after the rite. Your share might go something like this:

> *Elder gods of forest and farm, city and wood, land and sky, this world and the other, [insert specific deity names here if you have them], I call you and pour out this drink in honor of you. May you receive it and may it strengthen our kinship.*
>
> *Great plant spirits of the green realm, givers of medicine and magic, harmony and rightness, ritual and beauty. Green beings who have their roots in the world of spirit and fruits in this world, [insert specific plant ally names here if you have them], I call you and pour out this drink in honor of you. May it strengthen our kinship.*
>
> *Good spirits of place, neighbors seen and unseen, guardians of this place and keepers of the ancient tracks, I call you and pour out this drink in honor of you. May it strengthen our kinship.*
>
> *To my ancestors three; those of my blood, this land, and the traditions I celebrate, I call you and pour out this drink in honor of you. May it strengthen our kinship.*

Finally, we participate in the rite ourselves and connect directly to the spirits by sharing in this sacred rite with them. We quite literally *take in* the power of the connection by drinking and eating with them.

> *With all my good kin I share in this sacred meal, taking this drink, I drink to our kinship!*

If you are celebrating with other humans, make sure that each person is given a sip of the drink before exhausting it. If you have companion animals who join the rite, a few drops can be sprinkled on their heads either as celebrants alongside you at the end or as an offering during the portion set aside for the spirits of place, to which our companion animals do have a connection.

Now, move on to sharing in the food portion of the shared meal. As a reminder, we do not bring metal tools into our ritual space, unless they are of soft verdigris metals such as copper or bronze. For this reason, cut out enough portions of the offering in advance.

Placing a piece of the bread at the base of the tree or into the offering bowl in the same manner we poured the libations, you may recite something like this:

> *Elder gods of forest and farm, city and wood, land and sky, this world and the other, [insert specific god names here if you have them], I call you and break this bread in honor of you. May it strengthen our kinship.*
>
> *Great plant spirits of the green realm, givers of medicine and magic, ritual and beauty. Great green beings who have their roots in the world of spirit and fruits in this world, [insert specific plant ally names here if you have them], I call you and break this bread in honor of you. May it strengthen our kinship.*
>
> *Good spirits of place, neighbors seen and unseen, guardians of this place and keepers of the ancient tracks, I call you and break this bread in honor of you. May it strengthen our kinship.*
>
> *To my ancestors three; those of my blood, this land, and the traditions I celebrate, I call you and break this bread in honor of you. May it strengthen our kinship.*
>
> *With all my good kin I share in this sacred meal, taking this bread I eat to our kinship!*

With the sacred meal shared, it's a good time to sit and soak in the experience. The spirits are often very present at these times, and if we create space to quiet down and enter into receptivity, we can receive guidance and inspiration directly from them. Spend as much time as you need. Once you've gotten good at this skill you can incorporate it into your monthly full moon rites as a way to add communication to the shared meal. When you're finished with your rite, appreciate the spirits for sharing in the rite with you by addressing specific points of gratitude rather than a simple 'thank you', which by tradition is considered dismissive. The candle and incense can be put out or left to finish if they can be safely left alone.

As a monthly celebration at the full moon, this simple rite has cumulative effects. Over time you will find that the space itself becomes charged with the presence of spiritual allies and the ways in which they start to show up in your life increases. These monthly meetings, when performed with regularity and passion, act as a keystone to our everyday connections to the deities, the plants, and our ancestors.

RAISING THE HEDGE

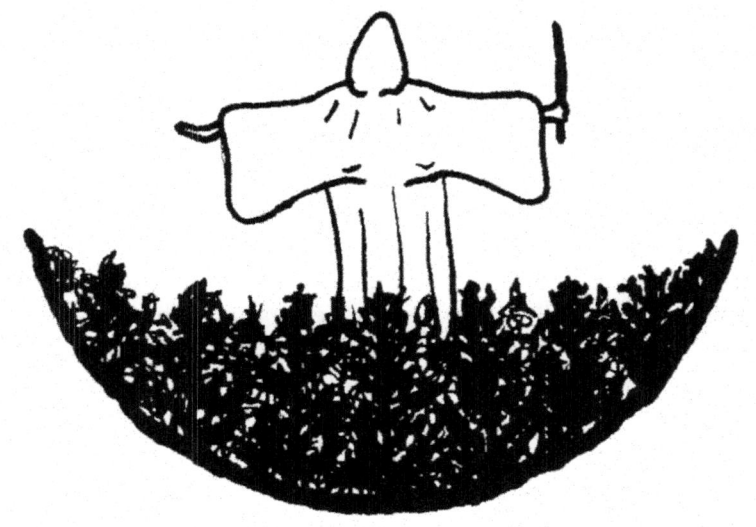

The hedgerow is an ancient symbol of boundary, protection, and defense. In the next chapter we'll be looking at one of the most crucial aspects of working with the plant sprits; journeying by spirit into their green realm. But before our journey, we are best served by learning to protect and deflect as a means to make our spiritual travels safe and effective.

Raising the hedge is a simple, imaginal process of growing a circle, as large or small as you want it to be, of protective plants or verdant green light all around you. You can do this indoors or out, and you have full creative license over how it's done, and which plant allies are called into the process, if any. In my own work I raise a massive hedge of Privet (*Ligustrum vulgare*), a common shrub used as a natural fencing, to surround me. I focus on their roots extending deep into the earth below me and their sharp-thorned branches growing high up into the sky around me. I generally begin by imagining the circle itself, then use my inner vision to grow the hedge from seed to sprout to great wall of green. You can work with any specific plant or plants you feel carry a protective energy for you or simply call in a powerful green light.

Protection

There are very real reasons to encircle yourself in a hedge of protection when doing journeywork or rituals. Not all the spirits who share space with us are happy about it, and our workings can sometimes attract the attention of unwanted guests. The simple act of raising a hedge is powerful as a working of energy magic, but more importantly it acts as a visionary petition to the plant spirits all. When we raise the hedge, the verdant power is with us and we are surrounded by the protective energy of green and the plant spirits we're allied to.

Letting go

For many of us, especially folks who have dealt with trauma, anxiety, and fears, the idea of letting go for flights of the spirit can be frightening. Raising the hedge is a powerful and therapeutic way to find peace and safety in the spaces you choose to create for yourself. The sovereignty that this practice builds is real, and in time it trains us how to fully inhabit, with respect, the spaces we live in.

The more our fears and mental chatter can be quieted, the easier our travels and the further in we can go.

The body

Since we are leaving our physical guard down to some degree, a layer of protection for the physical body is another benefit to raising the hedge. It helps to secure the level of the physical form while we travel in spirit flight.

Deflection

The nature of trees and plants is that they absorb and transmute many energies, namely that of the sun. In a similar way, when called to the hedge they can help to deflect and transmute any negative, harmful, or toxic energies from within or around the circle during our work. As we excel at this practice, it becomes a ritual of healing in and of itself. Surrounded in green and by the presence of our protective allies, energies and patterns are taken from toxic states and composted into neutrality or beneficence.

Allies of protection

You can work with any specific protective plants for this practice, or a non-descript green protective presence of light. Over time, I encourage you to call in one or several of the plant spirit allies you become close with to ask their special support in raising your hedge. You'll find the efficacy and mood of the hedge changes dramatically when you know the allies standing guard for you.

Raising the hedge

To open your own sacred space and surround it with deep green protection:

- Pace or otherwise mark the space you want to protect. This should be enough for you to feel comfortable but not so excessive that you feel you're in an empty room.
- Take your ritual position, which could be sitting upright in a chair, laying on your back, or even standing upright. From here, imagine the hedge growing up all around you from seed to sprout, small shrub to massive hedge. If working with green light, begin with a line and slowly expand it to surround you.
- Experience the towering presence of the plants above you reaching far into the sky and their expansive root system reaching below you. Feel yourself wrapped in a cocoon of safety and security.
- I often experience a vortex of vibrant green light swirling around and through the hedge once it's constructed.

- When your work is done, draw the hedge back into the land in reverse order: hedge to shrub, sprout to seed. Experience the space returning to usual. You can pace the area once more to reclaim it or to disperse any lingering charge of energy, if you feel inclined.

A hegde of protection

Take time to practice, experiment, and learn the ways of hedge raising. Think about which plants or trees call up feelings of protection and security for you. Consider plants with thorns, those that grow densely, or those with tall, imposing features. Explore different ways to raise the hedge with your inner vision, then challenge the strength of it by pacing the perimeter and pushing your palms against it or passing your arm through it. How can you make your hedge stronger, thicker, taller, or more secure feeling?

A MAP TO THE GREEN REALM

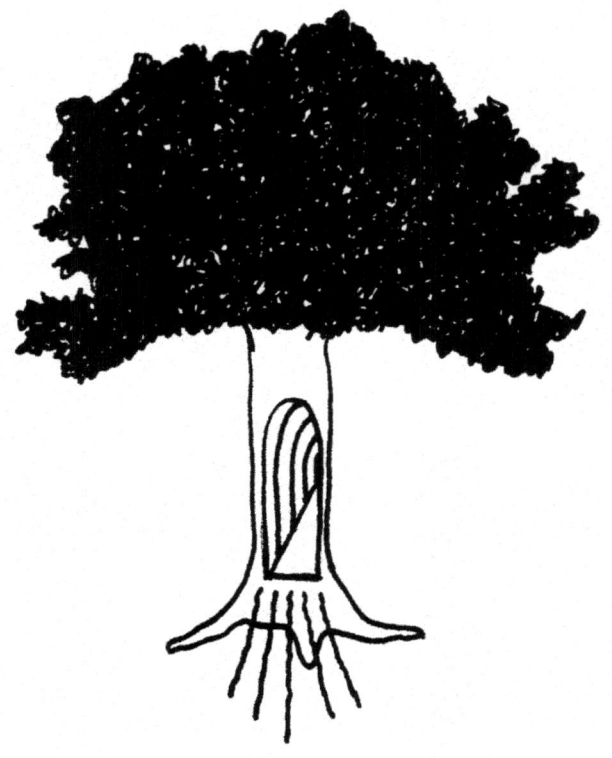

It is a foundational arte within all the world's visionary-animist traditions to journey by spirit into the realms of otherness. By learning and strengthening this skill, we're able to cultivate relationships of sorcery with our spiritual allies to gain wisdom, guidance, and initiation that speaks directly to each of us. These methods are the very same that have allowed the herbwise of old to learn from the plant spirits and write down what was to become the celebrated materia of many traditions.

We're able to engage with the world of spirit because that world saturates our own. While separations exist, there is a fundamental unity which allows access to the adept of what we call *spirit flight*. In this work the inner faculties of spiritual vision, our ability to see with the mind's eye, allows us to reach out and connect with the green realm to explore and relate in power. The imaginal realm within becomes a meeting place where our world and our own language symbols dovetail with those of the plant spirits, elder deities, land spirits, and ancestors. Here we can openly communicate with people and places that are distinctly *other* to our own, all while sitting comfortably on our living room floor.

In this chapter we'll explore a simple way to journey to the green realm where we can have direct, personal experiences with otherness and all its varied inhabitants.

Plant spirit liminality

As we embark on our work of spirit flight, we are well served to remember that the plants are always there to help us on our journeys. They can do this in two ways. First, they can help us move through the hedge that usually separates our world from the otherworld by giving us special guidance, protection, and access to these sacred spaces. Second, they can be worked with in more physical ways in the form of salves, oils, and balms to help drop us into altered states of consciousness while brightening the spiritual vision within. Look for a salve, oil, and tea in the grammar section to help you take flight.

The tree at the crossroads

Keep in mind the symbolism of the tree. In the work of spirit flight, the tree acts as a crossroads where we can access other realms, worlds, and perspectives for our spiritual development. When we journey, we begin by passing through a tree doorway, which transports us to the realm we seek to explore.

In this map, we work with the Oak tree. This tree ally carries the virtues of a gatekeeper and has been a guide into the otherworld since ancient times. The old Irish name for Oak, Duir, is where we get our modern word *door*. The Oak was once held so scared for this work that we see the genus *Quercus* in the modern word *church*. You are encouraged to work with any strong plant ally you have as a doorway to the green realm, as all plants and trees may help you to do so, but initially try working with Oak as they're exceptionally willing to aid us in spirit flight.

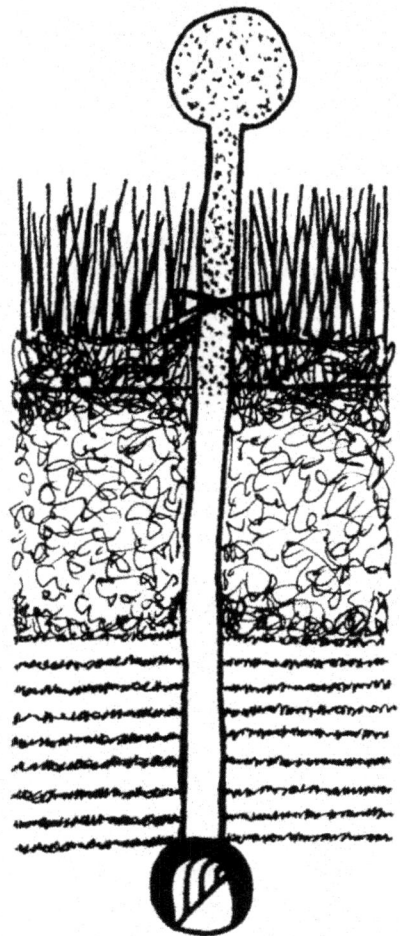

The map

The map I work with to journey to the green realm is simple. Each presentation of symbolism has important meaning and function. For now, I invite you to follow the map as it is—but be aware that over time your own shall develop.

The map allows several things to happen. First, it brings us into a gently altered state of consciousness where it becomes easier to interact with the otherworld and its inhabitants. Second, it activates our faculties of inner vision while quieting our usual physical senses, so that we can fully engage on a spiritual level. Finally, it gives us a clear and reliable path in, around, and back out safely.

Following the map is a lot like taking a guided pathworking or creative visualization. You'll be given symbolic cues to work with, at your own pace and with a great deal of creative license, so that you can reach through the hedge and explore.

Before we get started, I would like to give you two important considerations. First, no matter how you venture into the green realm, always come back the same way you went in. Second, do not eat or drink anything when in the green realm. This is a taboo of our tradition and one we will explore in more detail later on.

Begin your journey ...

- Create a safe, comfortable, and quiet space for yourself where you can be free from distractions and disturbances. Some light ambient background music, white noise, or drumming can be used if those things are helpful in quieting body and mind. You can also light a candle and burn some botanical incense to set the space if you like.
- Start by raising the hedge to ensure your body stays protected and your journey is surrounded with safety.
- Settle into a seated position on the floor or on a cushion or small stool. I always teach spirit flight sitting up to activate the proprioception and to avoid people falling asleep.
- Do two or three minutes of green breathing to help quiet the nervous system, settle the body, soften the mind, and darken the senses. Allow yourself to drop into a comfortable trance state or altered state of consciousness.
- With gently closed eyes, call forth the image of a mighty Oak tree in front of you. Petition the Oak spirit to open a doorway for you that will give you access to the green realm where you can venture safely and return safely. You might say something like this:

> *Mighty Oak, doorway of the worlds, I ask safe passage as I travel to the green realm to meet my allies. I ask you give me entry to the otherworld and keep the door for me that I might travel back in wholeness with all given blessings in my keep.*

- Allow a doorway, portal, opening, or other point of entry to appear on the Oak in your mind's eye however it does. Whatever comes up is right for you and your own language symbol and should be accepted as meaningful.
- From the open door, a deep green mist which is self-illuminated pours forth and sheds light on a path that connects you to the tree. Walk, fly, float, or otherwise travel down this path intentionally. As you come to the door, be aware of the threshold and pass through it. Try to feel a difference between the atmosphere of where you stand now and that within the doorway.
- Once inside, you stand at a crossroads. Within the tree you are in contact with all the worlds and can call forth an engagement with the green realm.
- As the green mist lifts, you find yourself standing at the head of a long path which leads through three distinct spaces ...
- First, you move swiftly down the path through row after row of grain, which stands tall and strong, glowing gold in the bright sunshine. As you pass each row, the sound mimics a drumbeat which lulls you deeper and deeper into trance. This space represents our world—cultivated and controlled.
- The rows of grain then give way to an expansive meadow filled with fragrant flowers of every color imaginable. You can see endlessly in all directions. Moving down the path through the meadow creates a dull hum that lulls you deeper and deeper into trance. This space represents the wild places, which are approachable and comfortable.
- You then come to a hedgerow that borders an ancient forest. The trees are tall and mighty, and as you move swiftly down the path that takes you into the forest, it becomes darker and more mysterious. Although the forest is dark and still, you are guided safely down the path as if drawn in by an invisible force. The sound of the trees rushing by creates a combination of a drumbeat and a whooshing sound, lulling you deeper and deeper into trance. This space represents the wild, unknown, other.
- Soon, you come to a clearing in this ancient forest. You may find a fire pit, world tree, pillar, altar, or other item in the center, or the clearing may be empty save for the powder-fine dust on the ground, which has been trodden on by the herbwise folk who have visited this place since time immemorial.

- From here, the journey belongs to you. Invoke specific plant spirits to join you, call on the old gods of our ways, or simply explore and see where things go.
- The green realm will appear to you as it will, the plant spirits will show themselves to you in ways that work for you both, and other experiences will unfold in a language that speaks to your own heart. You may find the first many visits to be dull, colorless or monochromatic, lifeless, stagnant, silent, or confusing. With continued effort and return the realm will begin to show itself to you in fullness, along with its many mysteries.
- Remember well the taboos while in the otherworld. You are a guest, eat nothing, take nothing that isn't offered you and be clear what the price for it is, carry no weapons, and always express sincere gratitude.
- When done, return in fast-forward the same way you came in making sure to leave no trace. I find that coming out backwards so that I can watch the scene disappear behind me until I return to my physical body and usual state of consciousness is quite helpful.
- Spend a few moments stretching, tapping, massaging, and engaging visually with your surroundings to help with reintegration.
- Immediately journal about your experiences as you are likely to forget details from spirit flight in the same way details of dreams disappear when we wake.

Wortriding

Another powerful way to journey into the green realm is by working directly with a plant spirit who you have a close relationship to. Wortriding, as the name implies, is a method by which we visualize ourselves being carried on the trunk, stem, leaf, flower, or spirit of a plant into the otherworld. This is a powerful way to explore our own land and see how it appears from a more spiritual perspective, and an interesting way to move about in the green realm.

To work with wortriding, I suggest holding a piece of the plant in your hands during the journey. Raise your hedge, do some green breathing specifically with the plant ally you're riding, then close your eyes and call their form into your inner vision. Imagine riding or being carried by them into the worlds of otherness—even letting them guide you to places yet unexplored.

Your plant ally will carry you back to your body after the journey in the same way you'd return if you were doing a map-based spirit flight.

Gateway gods

Within every Animist, Pagan tradition we find gods, deities, heroes, or warriors who are celebrated as being gatekeepers. These gods have influence over both how the gates between this world and the next are managed and who ultimately gets through them. There are countless deities who manage their access to the gates in unique ways, so exploring who's out there can be quite a fascinating experience. These deities, after having established a relationship with them, can be asked to help you journey into the green realm and even guide or teach you while you're there.

The best way to meet possible gateway gods that might work with you is to look at the lore. See who shows up in myths and legends as a deity that gets people from one place to another, transforms them from one state to another, or has a dual influence over two contrasted spaces. Some general examples include the Irish Manannan, the Greek Hermes, Pan, and Hecate, the Norse Heimdallr, and the Gaulish Cernunnos among many countless others. You can work the lore to explore the personalities of these gods, see if you share any common interests, or simply see who feels the most attracting to you. When first starting, feel free to reach out to the great evergreen forest god, The Green Man, patron of the green arte tradition.

The relationship you cultivate with any of the old wild gods can unfold with meditations and prayers, study, and eventually ritual and offerings if things feel right. These gods, allied to us, can be called upon or invoked before we take flight to help open the ways and keep us safe in body and spirit during our journeys.

Magic and medicine from the roots

When working in the green realm, all actions, rituals, exchanges, blessings, and initiations shared have a very real presence back at home in our world. You will find that what is done in the green realm causes profound transformations here. They can be slow and quiet, but there is always a sense that a mountain is somehow being moved.

There is obvious caution to be given here. Be careful what you do and what you ask for.

INVOKING THE PLANT SPIRITS

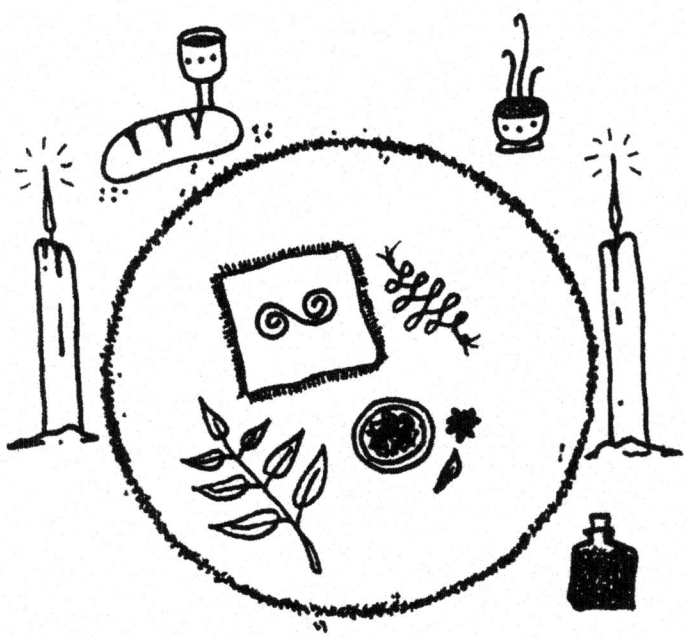

As we go deeper into our work with the plant spirits, there are times when we will want to invoke them to be present in our sacred spaces, at our rites, or at our working tables. We do this to ask their blessings on medicines made from their virtues, magics weaved with their power, journeys taken with their guidance, or dedications done in their honor. Invocations are a way to focus on the plant spirit, whether we're able to be with them in person as they grow in the soil or not, and it is fundamental to taking our medicine and magic work to new levels of potency and potential. Through this process we call on the spirit of the plant to infuse their virtues into whatever it is we are crafting; or to be present with us in a more tangible way for our communication.

We will be exploring ways to work with invocations later in the book, but for now I'd like you to have this information so you can contemplate it and know how it dovetails with later workings when we get to them.

What you'll need

- A candle: green is always an appropriate color as are natural beeswax tapers.
- Botanical incense (optional).
- Offerings for the plant spirit: food, drink, incense, etc.
- A representation of the plant spirit. If you are with them as they grow in the soil, then the plant themselves can be worked with. If not, you'll want something that holds the energy of that spirit. Possibilities include a jar of their dried plant material, a drawing or icon of the plant, a tincture or syrup made from them, incense of the plant where appropriate, written symbols or names of the plant that have significance for you, or a spirit house previously dedicated to that plant spirit.
- A way to mark sacred space. This should be a circle around nine inches in diameter drawn with chalk, flour, grains, dried flowers, meal, a line drawn in the soil, small stones, twigs, leaves, or other materials. Adjust the size of your invocation circle as needed for the space you have and what needs to go inside of it. If you are working with the plant in person, this circle can be drawn on the soil in front of the plant. Do not circle the plant form as this can feel entrapping to them. If you are working with a representation of the plant or a vessel of the spirit, that can be placed just outside the circle opposite where you're sitting.
- A bell, rattle, drum, or other sound maker (optional).
- The physical item or items you'll be invoking plant spirit blessings into. As we'll explore later, this might be a sachet, a tea blend, a tincture, a spirit house, or even a piece of meaningful jewelry that connects you to this specific plant person.

Once you have your items arranged, get comfortable and make sure that everything you need is within reach. This ritual can be performed anywhere you feel safe and sacred, but in the presence of either the plant themselves or a strong tree makes the experience much more powerful. Raise a hedge for added protection.

Draw or construct your working circle. I like to make my circle just a bit bigger than whatever goes inside so that it doesn't feel too constricted but also doesn't look awkwardly empty. The circle should be drawn in a clockwise motion while contemplating the cyclical ways of the plants: seasons, growing cycles, flower and fruits, seeds and roots, the sun and moon and earth. In essence, this small sacred space acts to part the hedge so that we can perceive the presence of the spirits in our work; it is an open portal to the green realm and a sorcerous act of great potency.

Begin the invocation ritual by lighting the candle and setting the incense in honor of the plant spirits in general and the spirit you're working with in specific. See the candle as a light to call in the plant spirit and the incense as a medium by which we make the atmosphere suitable for their presence. These should be placed just outside the circle to either side.

Place the item you are working on in the center of the drawn circle. If you feel some cleansing or blessing is in order, pass the item through light of candle and smoke of a purifying incense. I work with Juniper (*Juniperus* spp.) for this as they're an accessible tree where I live. If you aren't working on an item and are invoking the plant spirit for communication or journey, focus on their representative on the other side of the circle and their spirit condensing and becoming present within the seat of the circle.

From here, we connect to the plant spirit through the process of invocation. This is a deeply personal and totally unique experience for all of us. Here, we call out to the plant and ask them to join us where we sit and to bless us and our work by their virtues. You can write a poem or invocation in advance, make it up as you go along, add bell or drum, or even sing. It is your own emotional calling from the center of your being that acts as beacon to the spirits. If I wanted your attention, I might yell your name so that you could hear me—this works in our world. To call out to the spirits we need to lift our voices in a different kind of way.

I find a great deal of support and power in ringing a small, light-toned bell during my invocations. Not only are bells known in old Faery lore to attract the Gold Folk, they also help focus the mind, open the heart, cleanse the space, and make connections between the realms.

Place the offerings you have brought for the plant spirit next to the circle. If they're already there, touch them in acknowledgement of them being offered. You might be inspired to say something about the offering, why you chose it, and a petition to the plant spirit to accept it in kinship.

In this space, after a heartfelt invocation has been sent out, we drop into stillness and silence. You may work with any visionary techniques at this time to help you perceive the incoming presence of the plant spirit, or just sit and fully experience the space as it shifts. Each invocation may be different for you, and this is as it should be. Let the guiding presence of the plant spirit define the best way for the ritual to unfold. I will often use my inner vision to call forth a point or sphere of light which hovers just above the drawn circle. From there I let it shift and express however the incoming spirit guides it.

At this point you can begin your medicine making, magical working, journey, dedication, or other process. The invocation complements many of our magical and medicinal rituals as you'll see later on, so it's worth getting comfortable with this process. If making a tincture, for example, consider placing the empty jar in the center of the circle and adding the herbs, menstruum, and lid with intentional steps. If you're crafting a charm or amulet, the materials used can be assembled within the circle or placed there once they've been put together as part of the greater ritual flow. Always be aware of the presence of the plant spirit and in a mood of invocation as you do whatever crafting you do. Make plenty of space for the plant spirit to infuse their virtues in your work.

Once the working is done, the plant spirit is offered specific gratitude. We avoid saying dismissive or convenient things like 'thank you' and instead spend the energy to list specific things for which we are grateful—even if it is just that they heard our call and came to spend some time with us. The space is cleaned up, sacred items and tools are put away, and we go on about our journey.

This same rite can be used to invoke individual plant spirits, the plant spirits as a group, deities, or other good spirits with whom you are in good rapport.

INVOKING THE PLANT SPIRITS   121

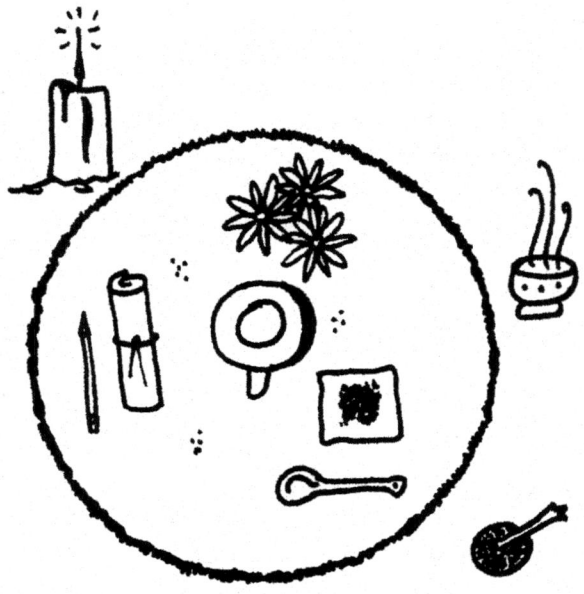

Beyond tea

I know we just looked at the process of invocation, but it's already time to experience it for yourself! Too often in this work we get stuck in our heads, find it daunting, wait until things are 'just right', or get hung up on the details of something new. Here's an opportunity to avoid all of that and just dig right in. I want you to experience this firsthand in a simple and straightforward way so that you can see just how approachable and organic plant spirit work can be.

In this practice you will go through the full invocation and participate in a powerful medicine ritual. My hope is that you will find this a beautiful experience and use it from here on out whenever you feel it's appropriate.

Here's what you'll need

- A large pinch of rice, dried corn, flour, slice of bread, or other simple organic material suitable as an offering.
- A candle.

- Incense (optional).
- A way to mark out your working circle.
- All the trappings for a cup of herbal tea, specifically: a cup, a single-herb tea (no blends for now) in a tea ball or tea bag, and a kettle with hot water. A simple Chamomile tea off the grocery store shelf is completely acceptable for this practice, as are a few leaves of Peppermint or a sprig of Rosemary from your garden.

In this invocation you will be calling in the plant spirit of the tea you chose and asking them to infuse the brew with *more* than just their physical virtues. If you have a specific reason why you're working with this ally, you can also ask for their helpful blessing on the tea as part of the invocation.

Using the outline above, draw the circle, set the incense and candle going, place your freshly steeped cup of tea in the center, state your invocation, and lay your offering near the circle with deep intention and power. Drop into quiet, tree-speed stillness as the tea steams and you listen from all parts of your being for the presence of the plant spirit. Once you feel they are even in the slightest way, share about why you chose them for tea, what you hope to learn and experience with them, and anything about them you are specifically grateful for. If you are new to this ally, don't ask for much just yet. Instead, focus on simply asking to get to know the plant spirit by having them infuse the tea with their deep spirit, virtues, and power.

Without hurry, enjoy your tea in the presence of the very plant spirit who indwells it. Follow each sip through your body, listen for guidance from within or without, see where your emotions and thoughts move, watch your body, and try to be fully present for this ritual of communion. When you're finished, continue on to offering gratitude and cleaning up. If you worked with flour, meal, flowers, or any other organic material for a circle, it can be offered back to the soil, into a compost, or strewn across a garden.

Congratulations! You have just come into direct contact with a plant spirit and have made a connection to them. How did it feel? Do you want to spend more time with this spirit in different ways? Do you feel like exploring different plant spirits? What might you change about the ritual flow to make it feel more your own?

PLANT SPIRIT DEDICATIONS

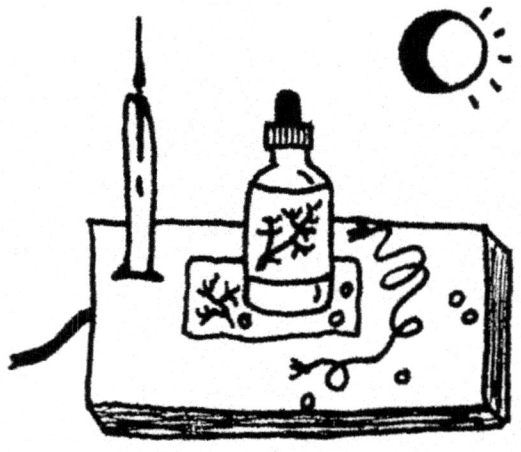

In the previous chapter you got to experience the presence of a plant spirit. Maybe you feel like you want to go further with them, or maybe you feel like a different plant would be a better match for you. The process of this work involves really being open to the many countless plants that share this world with us, doing journeywork to the green realm where we can meet spirits who want to work with us, and paying attention to the plants who show up on our path in everyday life. As we start to notice connections with specific plants, we honor that by giving them offerings of space and time in our lives for the relationship to unfold. Just like when we meet a new human friend, we invest ourselves in learning about them, letting them learn about us, and just sharing life together as we step into harmony within one another.

One of the most powerful ways to do this is through a plant spirit dedication. These are a lot of fun, incredibly interesting, and very effective at helping us learn the lore, virtues, traditions, and personalities of the plants. For my students, dedications are essential, and we spend weeks and months with individual plants to give plenty of time to get to know them. During this time, we all get powerful and personal inspirations from the plants we're dedicating to—often in ways we never expected. These dedications mark the beginning of plant spirit familiar relationships.

Here I offer you three paths to work a plant spirit dedication. They are each very similar in nature but differ in length and intensity. Before we get started, there are three things to consider. First, do you feel a connection or call to this plant? What makes you want to dedicate to them? Second, is this plant safe for you to consume internally or do they need to be worked with in a purely external way? Third, make absolute certain that you will finish what you start. We call these rituals *dedications* for a reason. We are dedicating, or offering, space and energy and time to the plant spirits. Once we begin the ritual it is of utmost importance that we finish it.

The plant spirit dedication is a way for us to carve out time in our busy schedules to just sit with the plant spirit we are working with. It gives us an excuse to unplug and quiet down and creates the right kind of atmosphere for deeper communication and sharing to happen. These experiences are unique to each human who enacts them and are often dramatically different from plant to plant, so prepare for the unexpected even after you've done these many times. There have been times that month after month my dedications were relatively similar only to have a new plant ally come in and make the journey so wild and diverse that I wasn't really sure what to expect from one day to the next. Those are, of course, my very favorite!

In our dedication work, we perform a simple beginning ritual to start the process. From there, we spend a bit of time each day interacting with the plant spirit with openness and intention. We also work to carry their energy with us throughout our whole day so that we can attune to them as much as possible. Dedications can be done in 3-, 9-, or 29-day lengths depending on what feels right. The 29-day lunar cycle dedication is the one that carries the most power, but when we're beginning the work sometimes the shorter lengths are a bit more manageable. Each of the 3, 9, or 29 days of our dedication gives us an opportunity to read lore and study about the medicinal or folk magic virtues of the plants, connect with them in nature or through photos, explore their anatomy and growing patterns, journey with them, meditate on them, take them as medicine if they are safe to do so, carry them on our person, dream with them, bathe in them, and offer a place of honor for them on our altar or shrine. You have complete creative license on how the process goes, and by the end of this book you'll have many different ways to fill the days.

For the sake of simplicity, we will assume that the plant you are working with is safe for you to take internally as medicine. If not, please make creative adjustments accordingly.

The 3-day dedication

This is a fantastic starting point when you are just beginning the work or when you are connecting to a plant that you feel called to but aren't sure just yet. Three days is a small sacrifice, and if for some reason things just don't feel the way you want, it's an easy length of time to make it through.

In our example, we will be working with Chamomile, who is a plant suitable for most people to work with internally and externally as desired.

DAY ONE

- Create a small altar or space on your shrine to the Chamomile spirit. Place a jar of dried Chamomile flowers, a printed photo of them, a fresh bundle in a vase, or some other representation. You might set this on a white or yellow cloth and keep a small vial of Chamomile essential oil and a Chamomile tincture there as well.
- We carry a small bit of the plant with us throughout the whole dedication; many of us even taking them to bed with us to help inspire dreamtime journeys. Prepare a small sachet sewn with dried Chamomile, a dried piece of root wrapped with a string of an appropriate color, or even a small vial of tincture that can be safely tucked in your pocket.
- Perform the invocation ritual from the last chapter with a focus on asking the Chamomile spirit to bless and empower the item, and any other relevant items to your dedication, as a link to them. You'll also want to use the working section of the invocation ritual to state your

intention to offer a 3-day dedication and ask the plant spirit to be with you. Carry the item with you all the time to stay in contact with the spirit. If you need to leave it behind, keep it on the altar space dedicated to this plant spirit.
- Set aside time to sit in communion with the plant spirit. Sip on Chamomile tea, take just a few drops of tincture, anoint pulse points with diluted essential oil, or hold fresh Chamomile flowers to your heart. This is a time to breathe, open, and listen. You can also take this time to journey to the green realm, invoke the Chamomile spirit there, and connect to them while having their medicine coursing through your physical body.
- Journal immediately after the experience so you remember everything that happened. These writings become your own green grammar, materia medica and magica, and sacred text.

DAY TWO

- Make priority time to sit with the plant spirit again; once or twice a day is fine, and these sessions can be as brief as ten minutes. Remember to journal about your experiences.
- I also encourage you to use this time to read up about the botany, medicinal virtues, magical virtues, lore, and legends surrounding your plant spirit. Get to know them!
- Carry the plant with you all day and find time to study and research lore, myth, and traditional ways this plant is worked with. Try to be mindful of their presence with you as you walk your path.

DAY THREE

- Once again carry the plant with you and make time to sit with them. Journal about your experiences
- At the end of this, our final day, enact a simple ritual of gratitude. You might consider making offerings to the plant spirit, reciting any poetry or lore you found for them, or just sitting with them one last time in contemplation and receptivity.
- Acknowledge the dedication as complete. You can keep any items you crafted on your altar or return them to the land if you feel so called. Tinctures and teas can be stored away for when they're needed in the future.

The 9-day dedication

In working a 9-day ritual, you can follow the same guidelines as the 3-day but with more time to get to know the plant spirit. Make sure to mark the first day with some sort of initiating ritual and the final day with gratitude and acknowledgement of the journey. At nine days you will experience quite a bit more about the plant than you might imagine, and you will create much more room for them to work their way into your heart and mind.

The 29-lunar cycle dedication

This is by far the most powerful way to dedicate to a single herb ally, and the method that requires the greatest amount of sacrifice. For those who are willing to do the work, I assure you that the rewards will far outweigh any frustrations you may encounter along the way.

In a lunar cycle dedication, we align to the tide of the moon and sit with a single plant spirit for right around 29 days, or whatever length the lunar cycle you work on happens to be. The rhythm set by following the moon allows us start with subtlety, peak with intensity, and end with a different type of subtlety. This is by far my favorite way to go in deep with the plant spirits and really get to know them and learn directly from them.

PREPARATION

Before you start, there are a few things you'll want to have on hand to make this rite one of depth and power.

- Journal or notebook with ample space for a whole month of writing and doodling.
- A standard tincture of the plant you are working with—in this case we are only working with plants that are safe and supportive for you to consume internally in very small doses.
- A square of cloth and a length of string to tie a small sachet. Ideally, choose colors that represent the plant you're working with.
- An ounce of two of the dried plant.
- A representation of the plant; photo, small glass jar filled with dried material, vase with fresh material, dried root piece, icon, or amulet.

- A candle to light during journeys and meditations. Beeswax is always preferred here. Consider rolling it in the dried and powdered plant to connect.
- Materia media, herb magic, and lore books or bookmarked websites that include entries for your focus plant.
- A small glass cup, shot glass, or port glass filled with clean water.
- Any other meaningful decorations, statues, or items you feel inspired to bring in.
- Optional items: A second length of colored string, oil or balm made from the plant, incense crafted from the plant, access to the plant as they grow in the soil, or tea to sip on throughout each day to keep the work going.

DAY ONE

We begin our journey at sunset on the evening after the new moon when the first sliver of light appears in the sky. This is a time of new beginnings, initiations, and growth—everything we hope to get from our dedication work. On day one we craft a small altar for the plant spirit we are dedicating to, placing a representation of the plant and all the items we've gathered in preparation. Begin by lighting the candle and setting incense if you choose, then making a statement of intent to the plant and expressing your commitment to sit with them for a full lunar cycle. This dedication is important and should only be promised if you are ready to show up and do the work. For those who are comfortable at this point, a full invocation rite can be performed to call in the plant spirit and ask blessings on the tincture, dried material, and sachet items. The small glass filled with water (or other drink) is placed on the altar as an offering and should be emptied and refilled every single day with love and gratitude. Other offerings you feel inspired to make throughout the month are great!

The medicine for day one is a single drop of tincture. Yes, just one drop! Today we start subtly just as the moon starts subtly. In order to do this, we have to settle in, slow down, and get very quiet. We are actively listening *from everywhere* as we follow the drop of tincture into our bodies. We stay mindful of the presence of the plant spirit and allow them to speak to us from within—or just lead us on a journey of quiet reflection for a few minutes.

Each day we will add one drop to our dosage until we meet the full moon which will be our highest dose day, generally 14 or 15 drops. From there we will begin decreasing our dosage by one drop a day until we come upon the dark moon and finish our dedication with a single drop just as we began.

While still in this sacred space, make a small sachet with the cloth, string, and dried herb. A large pinch tied up or sewn up in a piece of cloth allows you to carry the plant with you wherever your journey may go over the coming month. I suggest carrying them in your pocket and sleeping with them under your pillow at night. During your daily workings you can place the sachet on the altar you've made for the plant spirit. If you do a full invocation, the completed sachet can be set inside the circle to ask for special connection and blessings from the plant spirit.

Journal about any experiences or just about how your setup and start process went while it's all still fresh in your mind. Note each day how many drops of tincture you took. If you did anything extra such as enjoy tea, visit the plant in nature, or read up on any lore or medicinal virtues of the plant, note those as well.

Extinguish the candle until tomorrow and keep the sachet with you to maintain the conscious and subconscious connection to the plant spirit you are dedicating to.

DAY TWO—FULL MOON

Each day, spend time at your altar connecting with the plant, taking your medicine, and leaving a fresh drink offering. The more time you allow yourself to settle and quiet so that you can really follow the herb plant with you, the better! You can also do journeys to the green realm to connect with the plant directly on days when that feels right.

It's a great exercise during this whole month to spend a bit of time every single day studying up on the plant you are working with. Use books, teachers, online classes, and websites as resources but make sure that the information is quality. Simple internet searches about lore, myth, and folktales surrounding the plant, recipes, monographs, medicinal virtues, traditions of use, culinary uses, and magical virtues can all yield a wealth of information to help you get to know the plant better, and to learn from the experiences of others who have connected to this plant. I share some great books for doing this in the references section.

Remember that you add one drop of tincture each day so that you can come to know the different levels of this plant as you go along. Be mindful of where in your body the medicine moves, what organs or systems seem to be stimulated or relaxed, what comes up in your mind and emotions as you sit with the medicine, and what synchronicities come up during your day that seem related. You'll also want to note areas where the flow of medicinal energy seems to be blocked, restricted, or uncomfortable. All of this is the plant teaching you directly from within and all of it means something for your lifelong connection to this plant.

AT THE FULL MOON

On the full moon we will be taking our largest dose of tincture, usually 14 or 15 drops. I like to spend extra time on this night in communication with the plant spirit.

You may consider performing a special divination with them if you have a tool you like to use, or use the techniques shared earlier to journey to the green realm and meet with the plant spirit directly on this well-lit night. You might also offer a toast to the plant spirit whereby a libation is poured in honor of them and then a sip is taken by you in kinship. Later on, I'll introduce you to *the shared meal* ritual which you can work into your full moon dedication rite.

Remember that at the full moon the plant spirits and many other spirits are more present and perceivable in our realm. Make good use of this time in whatever ways feel appropriate to you.

Starting tomorrow we will begin reducing our daily tincture dose by one drop a day until we're back to just one drop. Don't forget to record your experiences in your journal.

FULL MOON—DARK MOON

Continue your dedication, reducing one drop of tincture each night until you're back to one which should be on or one day from the dark moon. As the tincture dose gets more and more subtle each day, it's an invitation to go deeper and deeper into your own self and into the voice of the plant spirit. You may find, as I do, that the smaller doses elicit the loudest responses from the plants, or you may find that the smaller doses really require a lot more of your attention. Whatever happens, remember that in these moments you are being led and taught by the plant spirit directly—this is *for you*.

DARK MOON

On the last day of our dedication, we express special gratitude to the plant spirit and open our journal to read everything written. This is a way to ground out the full journey and see just where we've been taken over the past month. It's amazing how much happens in such a short time!

The dedication has now been completed, and you can deconstruct the altar as part of your completion ritual. You may do something extra if you feel called, including another invocation, shared meal, or journey. The sachet you crafted can now live on your altar as a link to your time with this plant or returned to the earth or compost if that feels better. If you want to continue working with this plant, or any other plant you dedicate to, you may find the beginning of a general plant spirit altar coming to fruition. Here you can keep representations of all your closest plant allies, and later on I will show you how to craft altars and make vessels for the plant spirits to reside in on your altar space.

From here you can take a day or two of rest and personal reflection, then at the first light of the new moon begin a new journey with a new plant ally if you want!

THE FAMILIAR GREEN SPIRIT

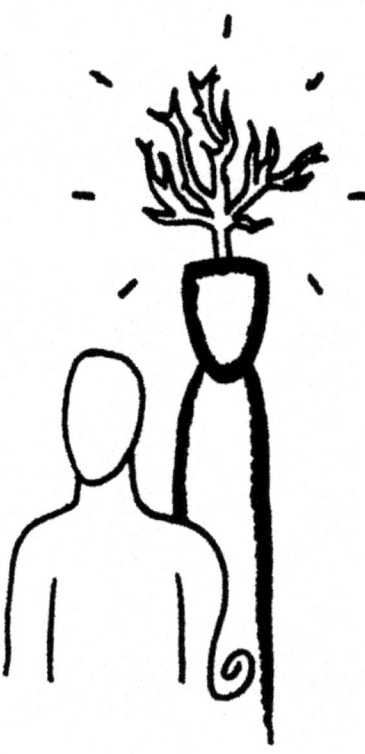

As you meet, study, communicate with, journey with, and dream about various individual plant spirits over time, it is the nature of this path that some will stand up and stand out as special to your arte. These plant spirits will be those who show up time and time again, speak the loudest, push you the furthest, heal you the deepest, and channel the most magic into your life. Sometimes they start slow and quiet, silent even, until you come to know them so well that their guidance resonates with you. Sometimes they roll in like a storm and shake everything to the core as they make room in your life for the medicine they bring. No matter how they come in and how they unfold, there is a deep knowing that the relationship is something special.

The familiar spirit is one who takes a personal interest in your growth, wellbeing, and contributions to the harmony of the world. Sometimes they have something in common with you such as an area of influence, what we might call 'hobbies and interests', or they might simply feel that they have blessings you could really benefit from. It also isn't uncommon for plants that seem *opposite* to us to become our most cherished allies—so never turn your back on whomever shows up for you. Their perspective allows them to see more of us than we usually see of ourselves, so even if the reason behind the connection isn't clear, it should be honored.

Over time, the depth of connection between you and your plant spirit familiar, or in some cases, familiars, becomes a central aspect to your work in the green arte. Our focus is always on sorcerous relationships that allow us to learn directly from the spirits- and it is the familiars who are most likely to impart the deepest and most powerful lessons to us as we walk down our paths. They come to know us as we come to know them and it allows for tailored, mentor-prentice type connections to blossom as trust and longevity are established. These spirits, true kin, become our verdant guides who give us access and empowerment to the wild old tracks.

Like any relationship, that of the familiar cannot be forced or rushed. It's friendship that crosses boundaries and that in and of itself is a magical thing. It takes extra work, extra mindfulness, and extra dedication to pass through this boundary and establish truly powerful working relationships. I wholeheartedly suggest that you focus on the journey and not the destination in this regard. Enjoy the process of learning, being seen, going on adventures of both spirit and life path, and everything that happens in between. This way your energy will be put in the right direction and the need to hurry or control the way things evolve will be released.

I bring all of this up now because I want you to have this type of connection to look forward to. I call all we do *work* because it is indeed work! The benefits are many, but the greatest is that we gain closeness to these beings of the otherworld and in so doing are blessed with wisdom, guidance, and power beyond expectation. Every bit of energy you put into your spiritual work is reciprocated.

Always remember that right relationships are the process *and* the goal.

SACRED FIRES

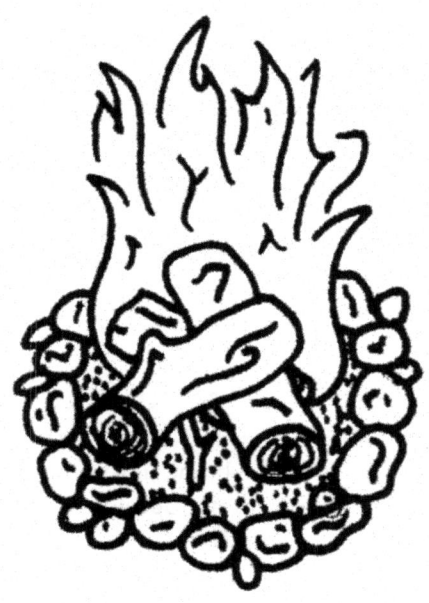

In all mystery traditions, fire is held as sacred. It is a bringer of light and warmth; lighting the path ahead and calling forth the vitalizing energies that keep us well on our way. In the green arte, fire maintains a special role in helping us keep shrine, open sacred space, honor our allies, and focus our efforts where they're most effective.

The need fire

In many tales from Ireland, Scotland, Britain, and other locales, a fire started with the use of flint and steel, rubbing sticks, or other hand-forged methods is considered superior. These fires were, and still are, often started as part of ritual observances or to honor contracts or taboos in a ceremonial context. The need fire, whose name comes from the idea that a central heart fire is quite necessary for both survival and to occupy a space, requires skill, effort, gratitude, and humility from the humans that seek to conjure it.

While there is no necessity to regularly kindle a need fire, it's a valuable skill to possess. Being able to start a ritual fire without the use of matches or lighter gives a feeling of empowerment and a special quality to the fire once it begins to roar. It's also a good skill to have just in case you're ever without fire starting tools.

If you've never started a fire by hand, I invite you to explore this magical working. See if there are methods that speak to you and try your hands at them. Once learned, you can utilize this method for special fête bonfires, to kindle the first fire in a hearth, or to honor your allies in outdoor rituals.

The fire of possession

In many European areas, we also find an observance that one has not fully taken possession of land or a home until a fire, usually a need fire, has been kindled in the hearth. In my opinion, this kindling speaks to more than just one's stewardship to a space. It symbolizes home and center, and implies that the spirits of place are being honored by the person who takes shelter there.

The fire of possession can be worked into many rituals. When outside, I often light a small pot fire or even a beeswax candle to assume the space, temporarily. I use this fire as a pact with the spirits of place that I will care for their land as my own and leave it at least as good as I found it, if not somehow better. The fire is a contract promising that for as long as the fire burns, I will take responsibility and accountability for my actions. Once extinguished, the area is returned in full to its inhabitants. This simple ritual of opening and closing an outdoor rite completely changes the feeling of the event and can open us up to profound support and blessings from the good spirits of place.

You can work a fire of possession into your rituals by adding it in to your hedge raising or to your invocations—wherever feels best to you.

Ritual fires

Our fires, from massive community bonfires to simple candles, create ambiance, direction, and vitality in our rituals. I find it important to have a living flame present in all my rituals, from simple prayers and meditations at my shrine, to larger outdoor celebrations of the seasonal fêtes.

There are many layers to the ritual fire, but two stand out as most important to me in our continued practice. First, the fire is an invocation. It both calls and can even represent the presence of deity in our observances and creates a welcoming atmosphere for all the invoked allies to enjoy. Second, there is a great deal of power in the reach of firelight.

The light cast by a ritual flame denotes sacred space. Intentionally or not, folks participating in ritual will tend to stay within the reach of the fire light and focus their work and energy therein. The flame kindled with intention and a whole-being connection to the work at hand acts as a further reinforcement of our grove and helps to generate more beauty and harmony. It can also be said that the light of our fire represents the area in life where we have the most influence or specialization. It is our family, our neighborhood, our communities, our cities, our professional groups, our social networks, and so on. These are the places where the work we do can have the greatest impact in creating positive change. While the axiom has always been 'think locally, act globally', more and more people are finding that taking personal responsibility for the well-being of their most immediate world allows them the greatest power of healing. The human and non-human people who live in our neighborhoods, the lands we walk every day, the cities and towns we call home, and our own social networks can well keep us busy if we simply take note of where we can be helpful. Healing and support are needed all around us right now, and if we all step up, suddenly more people are cared for than are not. In other words: the mountain, river, unhoused neighbor, animal shelter, food bank, mutual aid fund, and city council *that surround you* are your responsibility and would benefit greatly by your presence.

We will revisit fires when we come to the chapter on shrine and grove tending. For now, I invite you to connect and explore to all that fire symbolizes to you and means to your spiritual practices.

PLANT SPIRIT SHRINES

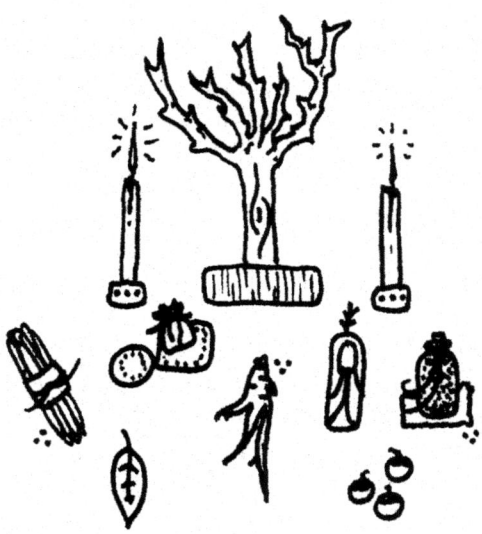

There is perhaps no better way to invite the plant spirits into your life than by dedicating a special space for them to call their own. Shrines allow us to carve out a bit of room, and energy, for the spirits to join us in more tangible and present ways—they help us to connect by engaging more of our senses and more of our everyday interactions.

Shrines need not be complex or fancy. They can be as simple as a cloth on top of a bookshelf, a small wood stand in a quiet corner, or part of a full working altar. Start small and let your sacred spaces evolve over time to meet you where you're at and work for whatever it is you end up using the space for.

Plant spirit shrines can be made two ways. The first is as a space to honor and interact with the plant spirits in general. The second is as a space to honor specific plant spirits, namely your plant spirit familiars. For most people who do this work, one space serves both purposes. This is a sacred point where you can honor the plant spirits all and those you are closest to specifically.

As a sacred place, the shrine is where you can leave offerings to the plant spirits, petition them, make medicine, craft magic, go on journeys of spirit, or just sit in quiet contemplation. The shrine should reflect you as a person and your relationship with the plants and plant spirit work. Over time, your familiars may even suggest or ask for things to be placed on the shrine to make it easier for them to work with you. Later, I'll be showing you how to craft plant spirit vessels and houses which make a powerful addition to your shrine.

Just a handful of uses for a plant spirit shrine include:

- To use as an entry point to the green realm
- To commune with the plant spirits and journey with them
- To place offerings and petitions in dedication to your relationships
- To put herbal medicines such as oils and tinctures while they macerate to honor the plants that invest their virtues into the medicine
- To craft sachets, incense blends, poppets, candles, amulets, baths, and more
- For divination
- To enter contemplative states more easily as you set in a pattern of use
- To acknowledge and participate in the changing of the seasons and the rhythm of the plant spirits in your area through décor and seasonal workings
- To provide a focal point for your plant spirit dedications

Items that are placed on your shrine should all be meaningful and intentional. If you are using the space to honor and connect with the green realm as a whole, you might want to consider what type of symbol would represent that for you. On my own shrine, a large carved wood tree stands for the world tree and is a representation of all the plant spirits and their otherworldly realm. I am also able to use this tree with its central knot as an entry point to the otherworld during journeys.

I also keep representations of the deities I work with, my ancestors as a whole, and the spirits of the land.

You might consider having some live plants growing on your shrine, if it's in a good spot for them. Many houseplants are quite happy to be part of sacred space and add energy to our work. They are, even when in pots, living bridges, making them a powerful guest in these spaces.

From there, representations, houses, vessels, or icons of your plant spirits or those you are working with at any given time can be added. You may have just one or two, or many. Over time the group who holds space on your shrine may change and adjust as you do, and this is both acceptable and normal for our work.

The shrine should include some type of offering at all times. A small wood dish and ceramic cup can hold offerings of food and drink, which should be replaced as needed. On my own shrine the spirits are fed every Friday and given libations of alcohol as it combines plant material with the ingenuity and labor of the human person, then fresh water the other days of the week. Again, the spirits will often guide you as to what offerings are appropriate to them, or you may be inspired as to what to offer them through lore or virtues. It goes without saying, I hope, that we are not the same people as our ancestors were and we do not use this space to bring harm or death to any animal. Bread made by hand or by someone local and good alcohol or fresh water are perfectly suitable offerings for who and when we are. Making offerings to the deities and your allied spirits is crucial to doing this work. We are given so very much, and it is part of the unspoken contract of sacred reciprocity that we give in return. While our gifts to the spirits need not always be material in nature, these should play a big part in our work since we are in bodies sustained by the physical.

I mentioned earlier that I replace a small bowl of food offerings on my shrine every Friday. You also might want to consider setting a day aside each week for special devotionals or meditations. I choose Friday for its traditional connection with the realm of Faery, which is very much aligned to the green realm. On this day the shrine is cleaned, old offerings are put in the compost bin, and fresh shelf-stable offerings are given to the spirits. These usually include bread, chocolate, local honey, dried or candied fruit, and other items that won't easily rot or attract insects. If you do make an offering of a more perishable food, allow it to stay on your shrine overnight or all day then remove and clean up.

Ultimately what you offer should have the work of human hands on it to make it special to the inhabitants of the otherworld. A flower plucked from your garden can be an appropriate offering to the deities or dead but doesn't work for the plant spirits. Food alternate offering ideas include song and poetry, salt dough creations, and watercolor paintings.

You may also want to dedicate a candle holder, incense burner, and small bell or chime. I like to ring a bell when calling in the spirits or making offerings to which they are quite responsive. I light a beeswax taper whenever I am mediating, journeying, making offerings, or doing any kind of work with the plant spirits along with some botanical incense as an offering. The candle can be put out between sessions and replaced as needed. Avoid candles with synthetic colors or fragrances—beeswax is always an effective offering and beautiful source of warm light.

Your shrine should be kept clean and organized. We find in much of the old lore that the spirits dislike clutter and dirtiness, especially in a space dedicated to them. Be mindful not to place anything on the shrine that you don't intend to consign to the spirits. This is not a place for car keys, wallets, or your water bottle.

One way to plan the layout and organization of your plant spirit shrine is this: how can you make it to be as much a reflection of what you experience when you journey to the green realm as possible? Are there ways you can make this shrine a physical map or icon of your experience of the green realm? This is a powerful way to create a shrine and make it relevant to your own personal work.

While your shrine design should be both personal and practical for the work you do, there is one symbol which I think is quite essential for the work: a representation of the world tree, center of the world, cosmic axis, universal spine. Your icon of the world tree could be a dried branch from a tree you're allied to, an artistic representation of a tree in wood, ceramic, or clay, a framed drawing hung on the wall behind your shrine, or even a living tree if you're adept at caring for small species and keeping them healthy and happy. This tree can be decorated with ribbons, ornaments, or symbols to mark the changing seasons and to align your shrine to the various energies of the year. On my own shrine, the tree sits at the central position and has in front of it a statue of the Green Man and images of plant spirits and ancestors to either side. I include a powerful ritual of opening for your world tree symbol in the grammar section.

One final note: don't start what you can't continue. Many folks get super excited about this work and dive in with big daily offerings and lots of workings. I encourage you to start small and simple. Consistency is crucial in this work as we see in the old lore and in our medicine experiences. It is better to pour clean tap water every morning for the spirits for years to come than to make grandiose offerings for a few months before leaving it altogether. In my own shrine service, I make clean water offerings daily and special food offerings once per week and at the full of the moon when I do more intensive workings. I keep it so simple that if I were to be in the throes of the worst flu or a broken leg, I could keep my commitments to the spirits as they keep theirs to me.

Later on, we'll explore alternative ways of shrine tending, and working with shrine spaces in the outdoors at groves.

PLANT SPIRIT VESSELS

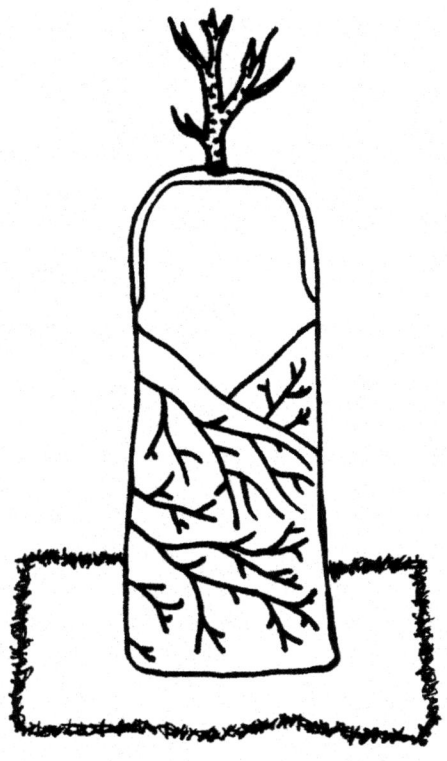

There is a practice within many of the sorcerous artes whereby a spirit is invoked and then sealed or otherwise trapped inside some sort of vessel or icon. This is probably the most pop-relevant reference we have to the work at hand, so I thought it wise to begin by saying that this is absolutely *not* what we do! The creation and blessing of plant spirit vessels is a way to give a tangible, physical form to our spiritual allies. They can use these spirit houses as a place to embody and indwell when they visit our shrines and join us in our work, but let it be made quite clear—they come and go as they please. We are not trying to catch, trap, or otherwise keep them in place for any reason. Consider your plant spirit vessels a guest house for the spirits and know that the door stays open and unlocked at all times.

With that note out of the way, we can explore how plant spirit vessels can become a powerful tool in your work. Vessels, also known as spirit houses or icons, are a physical form that is crafted specifically with a plant spirt in mind. They are made with appropriate materials, colors, designs, and symbols to be suitable for the spirit being worked with, and they are constructed with a great deal of love. The whole point of a spirit vessel is to be inviting and comfortable for the spirits, so we should keep this in mind throughout the whole process.

Once a vessel is created, it is 'opened' for the spirit via a simple rite of invocation with the vessel in the center of the working. I'll give you a sample ritual at the end of this chapter. The opened vessel now belongs to the spirit and should be kept in a place where the atmosphere is kept peaceful, given regular cleanings, and given offerings on a consistent basis. It is both unwise and inconsiderate to invite a spirit guest to your home only to ignore them—so please don't do that. Remember that a simple pouring of fresh water, lighting of a candle, or burning of incense can be enough as long as it's done with the right sentiment and dedicated consistency.

Vessels are best when they're crafted by your hand. If your inner critic just took an opportunity to remind you that you are in no way an artist, sculptor, or craftsperson of any merit, I understand! The good news is that the spirits are not looking for aesthetic perfection. They are looking for connection, presence, and things which come from our world in service of theirs. Your vessel could be as crude as crude gets by our standards of artistic beauty and still be of great value to the spirits. There are many materials you can explore when crafting vessels, and many ways you can use what you know about your plant allies coupled with your own creative inspirations to make something amazing. A plant spirit shrine that hums with the energy of several active vessels and workings is something powerful to experience.

As a general rule, I exclude metal, plastic, and sharp edges from my vessels. I consider comfort, organic feel, and relevant colors and materials when planning them out and then let them unfold from there. When in doubt, journey to the green realm and ask the spirit directly how best to craft a house for them.

Here are a few ideas for vessels to get your creative wheels spinning:

- Salt dough or air-dry terracotta clay can be used to make small icons, plaques, or forms that are meaningful and relevant. Consider adding some powdered herb to the dough before allowing it to set. A recipe for plant-infused salt dough can be found in the grammar. These also take up pigments really well, so the finished product can be stained with a strong tea made from the plant.
- Drawings of the plant can be affixed to a thin piece of wood with a small stand attached.
- Clear or colored glass bottles can be filled with dried plant material, ideally from all parts of the plant. Consider adding decorative markings or ties to the jar to add more of your energy to its construction.
- Wood from the plant or a tree can be carved into forms that link to how the plant spirit appears to you in journeywork.
- Bundles of short-cut dried twigs from the plant can be tied together with cloth.
- Gourds and other plant parts that are hollow and carveable when dried make for perfect house-like structures.
- Small wood boxes can be filled with plant material, drawings, written names, or other resonant materials. The outside should be marked in some way to distinguish this vessel from others you may end up with on your shrine.
- A vial of tincture or oil made from the plant can be used as a vessel. It can be decorated with symbols, ribbons, or cloth to make it more attractive. Once dedicated, it should not be used by anyone but the plant spirit.
- The crafty type can fashion small wood houses, huts, or structures inspired by connected cultural traditions. These can be painted or loaded with items that align to the plant spirit and then dedicated as a spirit house for them when they visit.
- Perhaps one of the simplest and most powerful vessels for any plant spirit is their dried root. This is not possible for all plants based on their anatomy, but for those with smaller root sizes it can be quite lovely. I suggest dressing the root in a bit of cloth or colored thread to add your energy to it before opening.

This is really just a small sampling of what's possible. Your creative inspiration is important here because it carries the energies that will attract, connect, and please the plant spirits.

Opening the plant spirit vessel

Opening the vessel is an act of consecration. It gives us an opportunity to call in the plant spirit and dedicate the vessel to them for their use. It also allows for a subtle yet powerful link to be established between the vessel and the green realm, the green realm and us. Once the vessel is dedicated it becomes a gateway in and of itself allowing for the plant spirits to reach more easily into our world in fullness. Similarly, it allows us to be more connected to the otherworld and to have an easier access to the green realm in all our workings.

I suggest performing this ritual outdoors near the plant as they grow in the soil or at an established working shrine if possible, during the bright moon, at sunrise or sunset. Opening a vessel at a time when the plant is at a peak in their growth cycle and is accessible in plant form where you live can also make this ritual extra special.

Here's a simple opening ritual you can work. Feel free to make adjustments as they feel right for you:

- Gather all the items you need for your vessel. If you've created something in advance that requires extra time and work, have it wrapped up in some cloth or paper. If you intend to build your vessel as part of this ritual, make sure you have all the supplies and tools you'll need at hand.
- Refer back to the chapter on plant spirit invocation and work this ritual in its entirety. When it comes time to place something in the circle, you can do so with your vessel. When the meditation or journey section comes up, this is where we will state our vessel opening. Here's an example of what you might say during this step:

> *Great plant spirit [say name here], I have crafted this house in your honor and have infused it with my love and respect for you. A space has been made on my shrine, a place of honor in my life, where this vessel will reside. The doors of this vessel are now open to you and only you, and I invite you to rest here whenever you desire it, and to join me whenever I call out to you. Through this vessel may our connection be clear, my offerings be accepted, and our kinship grow.*

- Offer your own specific words of gratitude to end the invocation ritual. Then, with great respect, place the vessel wherever you have set aside a place for it. I suggest keeping the offerings made with the vessel for a full day and night or making new ones to celebrate the opening of the vessel.

The vessel is now open, and it is linked to both the plant spirit and to the green realm.

A few things to note from my sample words above. First, we make it clear that this vessel is open to the specific plant spirit being invoked and *only* to them. You can also ask their protection on the vessel to keep it pure if you feel inclined. Second, we remind ourselves and commit to the spirit that they may come and go as they please. We do this in good faith and in contrast to the horrible way spirits have been treated by many practitioners over the ages. Sometimes they are weary of us, and so we make these statements to clarify our intentions with them. Finally, we acknowledge that the vessel is there for work to be done. We ask that it support our connection to the plant, our continued growth with them, and our evolving relationship of power.

Mark the full moon at which you do your opening ritual. This can be a time each year when you pay special honor to that plant spirit and celebrate your relationship and their virtues; a festival day of sorts.

If you ever find that it's time to close this vessel for any reason, this can easily be accomplished. I suggest performing a new invocation ritual with the vessel in the center of the circle. Once invoked, tell the plant spirit clearly and honestly that you are closing the vessel and why you choose to do this. Express specific gratitude for all that's been done while the vessel was open, then ask the spirit to sever their connection to it. Experience this happening. Once you feel the vessel has been uninhabited, deconstruct it in some way that isn't violent or aggressive. Empty out herbs, untie a thread, wash in cold water, or some other action of ending. Finish the invocation ritual and return the vessel to the earth, water, or to a compost bin.

PETITIONING THE PLANT SPIRITS

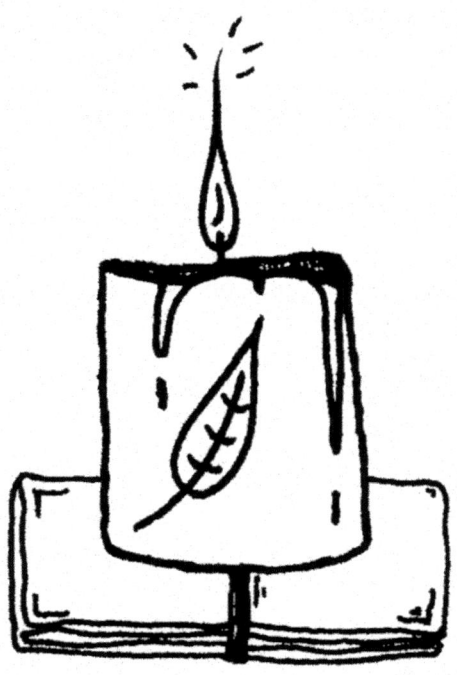

Petitions are a way for us to approach otherness and ask for what we need. They are requests made to the spirit world, prayers offered to the roots of our plant allies. Many folks, myself included, have a hard time asking for help or for what we know we really need in life. I value petition work because it helps me feel like I'm not just asking for things to be done on my behalf, but that I am showing up and participating in the change at hand.

Our petitions to the plant spirits are generally done with some ritual expression. This helps to get us out of our heads and into the world of nature, but also helps to ground out the blessings of the plant spirits in our everyday lives. Rituals create a space where we can try to meet the plants halfway and be as receptive and present for whatever they give as we are able. That being said, not all petitions need to have a complex ritual around them. The simple lighting of a shrine candle or offering of botanical incense can do as much as more involved processes. In my experience, no matter how simple or how complex the expression, we should *do* something. There needs to be an outpouring of energy to create space within for the plants to do their work. It is hard to fill a jar that is full, so our ritual expressions help to make room or shift things around so that transformation can occur.

An important point to consider as we explore petitioning work is that of transactional love. For most of us living in capitalist societies, it's easy to think of offerings and physical petitions as an exchange of 'I'll give you this so you'll give me that'. This couldn't be further from the truth of our work. Rather, as the Latin phrase rooted in ancient paganism goes, *do ut des*, 'I give so that you *may* give'. By giving, we are creating the space for blessings to come in. This is sacred reciprocity in action.

Another important point to remember in this work is that what we do is based on relationship. Where there is no relationship, it is generally considered inappropriate to ask for help. While many plant spirits will in fact step up and respond to petitions from humans they have no connection to, it is not in good form and often leads to dead ends in our greater spiritual journey. We should be willing to put the work in first—to step up and invest in the relationship for a good deal of time before we start asking for things. How long this will be is up to you, but for me it is not uncommon to suggest students wait a full year-and-a-day with an ally to begin petitionary work. Always remember how much the plants give to us every single day without fail. They have already given, so the invitation is there for us to meet them in the sacred cycle of reciprocity before asking for more.

So, how can we approach the plant spirits and ask for their help? Here are a few ways to consider:

- Your petition can be written on a piece of paper upon which a small beeswax candle is placed. Light the candle as an offering and beacon, connect to the plant spirits, and state your request. Small candles can be allowed to burn out with supervision, or larger candles can be put out and relit for some time each day.
- A physical representation of the petition can be crafted from clay, paper, or wood and placed on the shrine in the care of the spirits housed there.

- You can journey to the green realm and offer your petition to the plant spirit or spirits you're connected to. This can be a powerful experience as it opens the door for the spirits to respond and give you information about your request and how best to handle it.
- Petitions can be made along with weekly or full moon offerings, or as part of invocation rituals. This is best done with those spirits you have a longstanding relationship with.
- Petitions can be written on paper or organic cloth and gently tied to familiar trees or buried in the soil next to a plant ally. Be mindful that anything hung on a tree or buried in the soil won't cause any trouble for animals, plants, or the soil itself.
- A small pebble or stone found near the base of a familiar plant or tree can be charged with your petition and set down near their base.

As with all things in the green arte, your creativity is a powerful force in the work. What you feel inspired to do, and how you feel inspired to do it, often comes from the quiet voices of the plants. Listen, explore, feel, and see where the journey takes you.

In an upcoming chapter we will explore more potent forms of plant spirit magic. For now, I invite you to contemplate in your own way what the differences between *petitions* and *magic* are, if any. When we get to our section on magical workings we will be revisiting and building upon what we experienced here.

PLANT MEDICINE

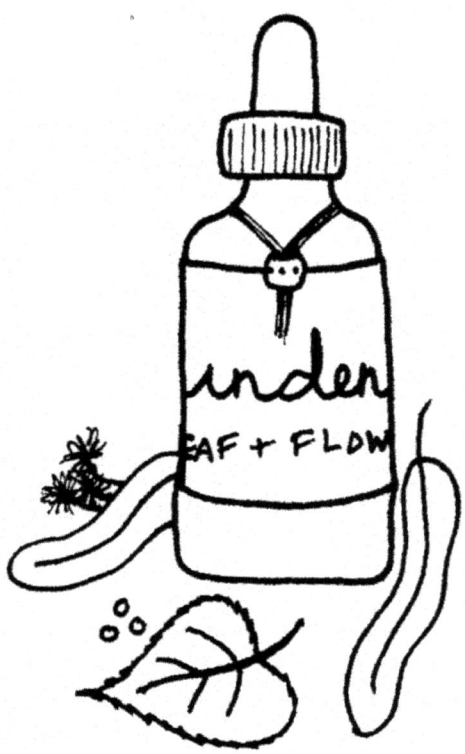

A book about working with the plant spirits would not be complete if we didn't mention one of their greatest boons to us human folk, medicine. The plants have always been our primary source of medicine and, I hope, will always continue to be celebrated, protected, and worked with to further our collective healing.

The paths that approach plant medicine mysteries are many, and although this diversity can be overwhelming, there is a common cord that unites the very best of them. This cord is woven from three threads: animism, energetics, and initiation. In this chapter I'd like to explore each of these three threads as a way to show you how I practice spiritual and energetic herbalism, and as an invitation for you to look at this work from a new angle if you're new to it or have been trained in a more allopathic and reductionist model.

Animism

This probably comes as no surprise by now. Those herbalists who practice their arte and craft with an actively animistic perspective will, as a side effect to that perspective, offer a deeper kind of medicine that is as much for the good of all as it is for the good of the individual being treated. Living in a world full of persons and especially acknowledging the plants as fully sovereign *people* changes how we approach the work. First, it ensures that our medicinal ways are in as much harmony with the whole of the living world as possible. It is good insurance against cultural appropriation, overharvesting, theft, and misrepresenting established herbal traditions; all of this being crucial to practicing good medicine. It also means that the way we see the herbs as medicine and the humans as recipients of that medicine will be dramatically different than those non-animist traditions that focus more on what the herbs are 'good for' and how they can be 'used'. The 'this herb for this disease' approach is one that is in stark opposition to truly spiritual herbalism, and it's a perspective that silences the intuition, dishonors the plant realm, and gives the human recipient only a fraction of the healing that's possible.

Animism invites us to experience and work with the plants as fully conscious, complex, and invested spiritual beings who bring personality, influence, and power to our herbalism. It lets us step away from the all-too-common reductionist way of approaching herbalism and into a world where plant, herbalist, and recipient are in a dynamic relationship—magical *and* medicinal.

Energetics

Also known as *constitutional* or *humoural* medicine in many of our ancient traditions, energetics is a way to explore more intimately the personalities and influences of the plant spirits. The language of energetics lets us discuss how an herb that has an affinity for the respiratory system does so in subtle nudges towards states that are almost completely overlooked by current forms of Western herbalism. A list of herbs that are *good for* the respiratory system tells us only a small part of the story of the plant spirits—and to reduce them in this way instantly cuts us off from the timeless magic that is plant medicine while offending their sovereignty and personhood.

Energetics gives us access to the subtle way that the herbs heal and a greater understanding of the human body and disease states. The whole practice of energetic herbalism is a constant, evolving meditation on healing that is dynamic and adaptogenic, as it meets every individual person we serve wherever they may be.

The energetics we most commonly work with in ancient traditions of herbalism, especially those from the West, are made up of four states that relate to body, herb, and element. Those energetic states are cold, dry, hot, and damp, which are connected to the four primordial elements of earth, air, fire, and water. Let's look at how an understanding of herbal energetics changes the mood of the work dramatically while also increasing the efficacy of our herbal preparations many times over.

In most herbal books, you might turn to a chapter on *herbs for the respiratory system* and find a list of ten or fifteen herbs with some cursory information about that they're *good for*. This herb is an expectorant, this herb soothes a sore throat, this herb relaxes the breathing, and this herb fights viral infections in the sinuses and upper respiratory system. Great! That's a fantastic beginning, but it's only a fraction of the real story. Energetics allow us to explore *how* the herbs do what they do when brought into our bodies. Mullein (*Verbascum thapsus*), for example, is a celebrated respiratory ally that helps to calm and clear the lungs through expectoration and thinning of mucosal build-up. But how? Mullein leaf is a *damp and cool* herb. They carry a powerful demulcent that, especially when taken as a tea, provides mucilage to the lungs to flush heat, coat tissues, break down and thin out stagnant phlegm, and allow easier expectoration without all the hacking and throat irritation. What if you didn't know this energetic of Mullein leaf and gave them to someone who was indeed struggling with a respiratory issue—but one that was incredibly wet, rattly, and phlegmy? You would be adding a damp respiratory herb to already damp lungs. While some relief is to be expected, the issue could get worse, could be driven further down into the lungs, could prolong the recovery, or could invite in other serious problems. What to do? Choose another respiratory herb with expectorant support that leans toward the *dry* energetic, such as Coltsfoot (*Tussilago farfara*) or Yerba Santa (*Eriodictyon* spp.). Dry respiratory herbs for a wet respiratory condition; the air element checking the water element.

For a more immersive study of this topic, I invite you to explore my book *Spiritual Herbalism—the Magic and Medicine of the Plants*.

Energetics refine our understanding of how herbs work, how they influence the body systems and organs that they have an affinity with, and help us to ensure we are taking the state of the human person we're working with into full account before throwing general herbs at them. Action categories such as demulcent, carminative, alterative, astringent, and adaptogen are a great way to narrow down which herbal allies we should be calling in; but that's just an initial step.

The study, exploration, and personal experience of herbal energetics is what takes our work with medicinal herbs to the next level and amplifies the efficacy of our medicinal work with herbs in our communities. Taking the time to discover the energetic aspects of herbal identities also demonstrates our eagerness to embrace all facets of plants beings and our desire to *know* them as best we can—which they surely appreciate.

Initiation

Who makes a human person an herbalist? Is it their herb school teacher? Years of book study? Successful support for clients? Published books? No, none of these things. The only authority who can rightly make someone an herbalist is the herbs themselves.. While all humans can and should have a connection to plant medicine, not all are called into the profession of herbalist from the plant spirits themselves. My definition of an herbalist is *one who knows the mysteries of the plants*.

Initiation means that we approach our learning and our experience from an angle that is in sharp contrast to how we usually consider learning in our modern world. The certificate at the end means nothing more than an acknowledgement of time invested and syllabus completed. Anyone can take a year-long online herbal program, but not all of them are really in touch with the spirit of the plants. Spiritual herbalism is distinct from other allopathic, reductionist, Western models of plant medicine in that the title isn't as important as the green blessings bestowed by the plant people.

It is only in our culture that we award people the title of *master herbalist* after just a few years of study. I cannot stand this term and wish I could erase it wherever it shows up. I have met one too many folks who are master herbalists after a 12-hour weekend seminar that have no real connection the plants, and certainly are not their masters. Another important point to consider here: where there is a master, there is a slave. Who is the slave to a master herbalist, and what does the master-slave relationship mentality say about the herbalist's way of working with the plants?

Initiation, for most of us, is hard-won. It is years, usually decades, of doing the work with the plant spirits before we are granted access to the profound mysteries of the green realm. It is study, exploration, experimentation, experience, ritual, dreams, disconnection, reconnection, and work done at the very root of who we are. It is joyful, painful, annoying, repetitive, uncomfortable, ecstatic, life-changing, and oftentimes outside our toolbox of expression. These initiations are gifted to those who show up and do the work. It comes in long, drawn-out waves over years and in instants that flash like lighting and seem to expand heart and mind to hold a new perspective and wisdom not previously available. The plants are people, they are real, and they are aware. Their world is also real and we are connected to it in our work. As we take sincere steps down ancient tracks, we are seen and responded to—even if things get very quiet from time to time.

In my opinion, it is these initiations that we should be seeking and petitioning for. We want the plant spirits themselves to become our allies, our familiars, and our teachers from beyond the hedge. While our human mentors, ritual guides, favorite books, and epic myths shine a special kind of warm light on the path, we walk it alone in the eerie presence of the green others. From there, it is what we provide our communities that define our position as herbalists with the blessings of the plant spirits as our living lineage. Relationships with the plant spirits is both the process and the goal of the spiritual herbalist.

Giving medicine

When medicine is handed from one who has a sincere connection to the plant spirits to someone who seeks that medicine, the power that has built up in the herbalist's relationship is carried through in the remedy to the recipient. This is incredibly important in our work because it means that *without* the intimate, hard-won relationships of plant spirit work, the medicines we craft only tell a small portion of the wisdom story. All the time, energy, study, experimentation, experience, and dedication to teachers and learning the herbalist has done will change the taste of the tincture, the brightness of the tea, and the depth of the oil. Relationships of the green arte should be the goal of folks who go beyond reductionist herbalism and enter into the wild world of herbal sorcery.

So, to summarize, herbalism is a spiritual practice that involves experiencing the plants as real beings who carry complex and powerful expressions of influence, and working with them to become steward for their medicine and magic in service of a community that acknowledges and engages with our work in an organic way. Spiritual herbalism is an approach to healing that honors the whole being of both human and plant—and calls upon one who can cross the hedge between their respective worlds in ritual, petition, and crafting. When our herbalism moves beyond recipes and reductionist lists of what an herb is *good for*, we ignite a lantern that both guides us down the old track and attracts the plant spirits themselves.

In the grammar you'll find a brief how-to that shares my way of crafting herbal tinctures. If you've ever done this before, I think you'll find some new perspectives and subtle ways of approach that take your tinctures beyond being just medicine and imbues them with magic.

TOOLS OF THE ARTE

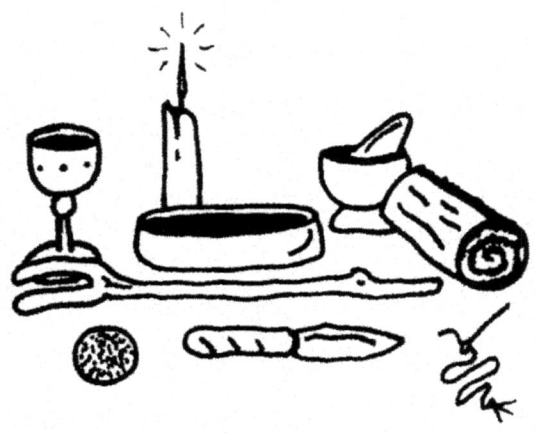

What is it about those of us called to more ritually-oriented paths that makes us swoon over tools? We do love to collect, make, trade, and dream about that next addition to shrine, working table, or harvesting bag!

Tools are a powerful part of the green arte. They become like extensions of ourselves, new ways to interact with the worlds of form and spirit to craft our magic and medicine. Each tool, over time, becomes saturated with the energy of intent and can even take on a kind of liminal presence that pulls us into states of trance just by holding them. Tools are sacred, personal, and should always have a defined purpose in our work. If it no longer serves, it's time to pass it on to the next person. If it continues to serve, it should be treated with all the respect and care due the greatest of sacred objects.

The tools that may come into your practice are relevant for you and should have meaning and symbolism that speaks to who you are and what you do. In this chapter, I'd like to share a bit about the tools I work with most in my own practice and hopefully inspire you with new ways of calling them in, working with them, and learning from them.

Mortar and pestle

Perhaps my most cherished of all tools, the mortar and pestle is one ancient tool that inspires daydreams of old-time apothecaries and ancient plant work done by the devotion of hand and heart.

I have several mortar and pestle sets, each with a different application in my work. The one that lives in my herbal apothecary is large, heavy, and crafted from solid granite. We use this one to break down herbs, grind incenses, and powder up formulas before capsuling them. We also have electric grinders for this job, but some situations call for the special energy that the mortar and pestle bring.

I have a smaller stone mortar and pestle that lives on my working table at home. This one is used to grind herbs for incense blends, sachets, smoking formulas, and strewing blends. It is my magical vessel, a cauldron of sorts into which one form of the plant is put only to emerge charged and changed through my grinding, meditation, incantations, and petitions.

I keep a small wood mortar and pestle on my main plant spirit shrine which represents my herbal tradition, medicine making ways, and the mystery of the world. In this way, the mortar represents the land, the womb, and the dark places from which we all emerge. The pestle represents the world tree or cosmic pillar, the phallus, and the light places that call us all into ourselves. The gyrating dance that happens whenever herbs are ground in a mortar and pestle is a meditation on the joining of masculine and feminine principles, land and sky. Throughout the year I adjust the position of the pestle to aim in the direction related to the current season: west for Autumn, north for Winter, east for Spring, and south for Summer.

Even when herbs don't need to be pulverized, I will often give them a few turns in the mortar and pestle as I mingle my energy and intention with them and open them up through grinding and invocation for the work to be done.

Wand

The wand is an ancient and evocative tool that works with the wood blessings of the plant spirits to extend our reach from this world into the other. Wands can be crafted from many woods, whichever one is chosen should be meaningful and close to you. The wand I work with most often is made from an Oak branch that was felled during a lightning storm. It was one of the first wooden tools I crafted from a raw, bark-robed branch down to a smooth and oil-treated piece.

Wands can be used to invoke the plant spirits, open up the gates between the worlds, project energy and intention into magical and medicinal workings, stir dry herbs, or send out petitions and prayers to the kindred. They are connected with the Green Man, protector of the land and lord of the plant spirits. Having once been filled with the vital force of the tree, they continue to be a direct link to the spirit of that tree and all their green blessings and virtues.

You'll find my wood wand balm recipe in the grammar, which can be used yearly on the anniversary of your wand's making or reception, or as-needed to hydrate and protect this sacred tool.

Bowl

A very simple yet very important tool in my work is the bowl or vessel. While bowls are about as commonplace around the house as anything, I think one should be set aside for our plant work. The bowl I work with has been part of my life since I was a child. My grandfather kept this turned-wood bowl on his dresser as a place for loose change and mints. After he passed, I was fortunate enough to receive it from my grandmother and felt it was a good fit as a working vessel.

The working bowl should be made from non-metallic materials; wood being ideal, ceramic being another great option although more fragile. This tool is used frequently to mix herbs, mingle and charge them with your energy during magical workings, store plant materials on the shrine during rituals, represent the sovereign land goddess, or be the repository of written petitions or charms.

I have found, as have many of my students, that with just a short amount of time working with the bowl it becomes an active gateway of liminal power.

Verdigris blade

Metal is a touchy subject in the green arte as I practice it. Generally, all hard, sharp, and especially ferrous metals are considered taboo in accordance with the old Faery lore and are kept away from ritual, altars, and shrines, and the plants themselves. It is taught in the ancient stories that most all of the spirits from the otherworld, plant spirits included, scatter in the presence of hard metals, are harmed by their presence, or shy from them due to their use in human wars and ecological destruction. Keep this in mind whenever you bring any tools into a ritual space or sacred outdoor setting.

All of that said, we can work with certain metal tools with great delicacy and propriety when needed. There will be times when wood must be sawed, plants much be pruned, clay must be scratched, and cords must be cut. It is during these times that we work with appropriate metals, namely those that will take on a *verdigris* patina over time including copper, brass, and bronze. These *softer* metals are less aggressive and don't carry the martial energy that iron and steel do. Regardless, they must be stored and worked with using great care.

First, the blade, scissors, or cutting tool should be kept wrapped in a dark-colored cloth and tied with ribbon at all times when not in use. They should then be stored in a toolbox, wooden box, or drawer away from the altar or shrine. If you have a working table, you can of course keep craft scissors, sewing needles, and awls on hand, but they should be given a box or drawer for storage and kept there when not in use. My own scissors, which get used on a daily basis, have a simple cloth pouch with a ribbon tie.

These softer metals cannot perform many of the heavy-duty tasks that their iron or steel counterparts can, so they must be used appropriately. They are best handled for softer plant cuttings and harvesting, etchings, cutting threads or small cords, or carving wax or soft clay.

My primary harvesting tool is made with a Hawthorn wood handle and a hand-forged bronze sickle blade. It can cut through pretty much anything with a bit of patience and accuracy and brings a softer and more gentle energy to the harvesting process. When it doesn't work, I keep a set of pruning shears in their carrying case with an additional wrap of a dark-blue cloth and ribbon to help with tougher or thicker plant cuttings.

Sewing kit

If you're like me, you'll find many occasions to sew up cloth. Sachets, herbal pillows, charms, pouches, and more all make for the perfect way to bring the plant spirits further into your everyday walk of magic. While sewing supplies tend to be pretty common and utilitarian, I have found great power in arranging a kit that is set aside just for my work with the plants.

My own kit contains sewing tools that I inherited from my grandparents alongside needles, threads, and embroidery tools that work well for what I do. I keep this small kit with my other ritual tools on a shelf under my workbench.

There is great magic in sewing, and it should be meditated on whenever we run thread through a needle. The act of binding two pieces of cloth, weaving a pattern, or sewing up herbs can be seen as a ritual of connection. As we sew, each loop and every knot can be infused with our goals of magic and medicine.

Incense urn

I work with incense a lot in my practice. Smoldering herbs on a hot charcoal is a powerful way to release their virtues into the atmosphere, send magic and medicine to the countless directions, make an offering to the deities, or change the energy of a space.

Urns should be made from heat-resistant material. A small bit of sand or ash can be kept in the bottom to make them safer and easier to handle when hot. My favorite incense urn is one of Tibetan craft and is made from copper. It has a chalice-like base with a perforated lid. I keep black sand in the cup portion so that charcoals can be placed on top without conducting too much heat into the metal. This also makes for easy burning of pure botanical stick incenses such as those from the Japanese, Tibetan, and Nepali incense traditions.

A side note about incense: they are not all crafted equally. Most of the stick incense we're accustomed to is filled with rubber, adhesives, salt peter, combustibles, and synthetic chemical fragrances. These should be avoided as they do not speak to or carry the plant virtues. Look for incense that is made from pure plant material, has no internal stick, and smells like burning plants when lit rather than intense fragrances. Shoyeido and Nippon Kodo are both famous incense houses from Japan that create high-quality and affordable botanical incenses, and Incienso de Santa Fe continues to be my favorite overall botanical incense made in Albuquerque, New Mexico.

Ritual cup and plate

During our more intimate rituals with the elder gods, plant spirits, and ancestors, we often share in food and drink to connect with them. I like having a cup and small plate set aside for these sacred shared feasts.

My ritual cup is actually a Scottish style *quaich*, a shallow two handled drinking vessel, which is perfect for the pouring of libations and drinking of a shared ritual spirit. This *cup of friendship* is meant to be used in toasts, and so it spoke to me to buy one from a Scottish artisan online. It is made from ceramic and holds about ten ounces of fluid—the perfect amount for a general libation to the kindred and a drink for myself and anyone else in ritual with me.

In a pinch, any nice cup from the kitchen can be brought into ritual but having one set aside for our work with the spirits is preferable. If you know your way around ceramics or wood, I think it would be very meaningful to craft the ritual cup yourself in whatever style you choose.

My plate is a small ceramic piece from an online artist that's been glazed with the image of the Green Man.

We will be exploring the drinking cup, plate, and offering bowl as we work with them in ritual a bit later.

Offering bowl

The offering bowl is a place to make offerings on the altar or shrine. During rituals of shared meal, the bowl can receive the drink and food that will be shared with the kindred spirits.

The offering bowl should be made from a material that can be easily cleaned. It should be stored upside down when not in use so that an empty offering bowl is never set on the altar or shrine.

When I am leaving offerings in the bowl overnight or for extended periods of time, I will often drape clean linen or cheesecloth over the bowl to keep it from attracting insects or curious cats.

When doing ritual outside, offerings can be poured or set directly on the land.

Offering blend

At all times in my backpack and in the glovebox of my car, I keep a small upcycled mints tin filled with a blend for offerings. This is a simple way to ensure I always have a gift for the spirits and never have to take without giving or miss an opportunity to connect more deeply with those I connect to. I am one known to pull over at the sight of a Juniper tree, one of my closest familiars, and having something on hand to offer as a gift of kinship is always a good thing.

A blend for offerings can be made from rice, popcorn kernels, incense resin, dried flowers, bits of dried fruit from last year's harvest, salt dough shapes, fragrant wood shavings, cuttings of your own hair, birdseed, barley, small glass beads, or other eco-affirming materials. Make sure what whatever goes in your tin would be suitable to leave in pretty much any outdoor environment since you never know where you'll be when you need it. I suggest avoiding materials like metal beads, seeds from invasive plants, essential oils, chocolate, plastic, or very potent herbs in your blend. Keep it simple and heartfelt. It is not the material value of the gift that means anything to the spirits, but the energy with which it is given. Remember that the material offering is a vehicle for the real gift.

Mantle

Ideally green in color, this cloth serves to surround us in the energy of the green realm, focus our senses, and even offer a shield of protection. Instead of a traditional hooded cloak, I use a large wrap that is vibrant green and screen-printed with the face of the Green Man. I put this wrap over my shoulders when meditating, doing ritual, journeying, and even teaching to keep green in my field. I will also gently wrap my head during journeywork to allow easier spirit flight.

The green mantle in whatever form it takes can be washed in strong herbal tea blends to imbue it with the virtues of specific plant allies. I suggest leaving it to air dry so that the powers of the plants can really weave themselves into the fabric. I share a protective mantle wash formula in the grammar.

Sounds

I have a small collection of brass and bronze bells, rattles, and drums, which I use for various fêtes and rituals. As a minimum, a small bell can be kept to ring when invoking the spirits and calling on the old deities to join our rites. Bells have powerful association with the *others* and help to thin the hedge that separates our world from theirs.

Divination tools

I think it safe to say that most of us have some form of divination we work with. Those tools, be they cards or staves, coins or cords, are sacred tools through and through. By them we are given a more tangible and less 'heady' access to the guidance of our allies and the natural world at large. They give us a peek into the subtle patterns at play and help us to communicate more definitively with our familiar spirits.

Later in the book I'll introduce you to a simple yet powerful stave divination system that has become the foundation of all my casting practices. If you pull cards, cast runes or ogham, cast lots, throw bones, or do any other kind of tool-based divination, make sure those tools have a special spot of honor at your altar or shrine.

With all tools, it's important to make some formal connection to them as is traditional in folk animist ways. I like to prepare a special herbal tea, oil, or incense that I can anoint, bathe, or wash the tool in depending on what's best for the material it's made out of. A few drops of my blood may be added to certain tools to connect us. The tool can also be held while you journey to the green realm, once there being presented in its spiritual form to your allies with a request for their blessings and empowerment.

MEDICINE, MAGIC, AND MYSTERY

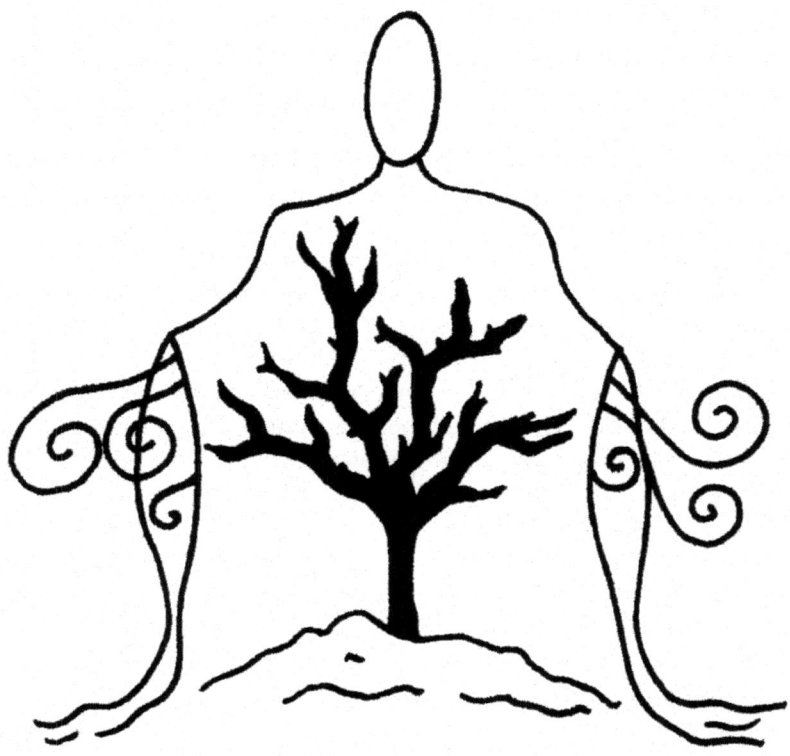

There are around 400,000 plant species on this planet that are known to science. That's a lot! In my herbal apothecary we work with about 300 on a regular basis, because we serve a wide community and many practitioners of many traditions and try to accommodate all the plants they love. In my own clinical practice, I work consistently with only about 20. In a world with so many plant allies, how do we learn their virtues, personalities, and spirits?

We have many ways of exploring the plants. From lore and legend to books and formulas, there is no shortage of material to sift through as we seek out our connections in the green realm. But how do we make this learning personal and meaningful? Anyone can open up a book on herbal medicine or herbal magic and see which herbs are 'good for' which situations, but as practitioners of a plant spirit path we aim to avoid the reductionism so common in modern plant spirit work and look deeper.

The plants show us their mysteries and virtues in many ways. First, their appearance is a direct expression of who they are on a spiritual level. The *doctrine of signatures* so crucial in the development of modern herbalism is all about reading the physical nature of the plant to glean information about their inner power. While the doctrine of signatures relies heavily on astrology and planetary symbolism, which is far outside my realm of knowledge, the idea of it works well for our purposes. We can consider the presence of a plant with our intuitive and analytical faculties to decipher how they might show up in our journeywork. A plant with stinging barbs could be seen as one with a connection to protection and defense. Plants with a sweet, attractive aroma might be associated with love. Those that bloom at night or grow in spirals might make us think of intuition, journeywork, and natural tides. Plants with pronounced toxicity can be allies in our exploration of death and the dark mysteries. Colors, bioregions, fragrance, patterns, and taste can all be assessed to make an initiation connection to a plant. From there, we connect to them in journey and communication to learn their spirits and research them in trusted materia medica to check their safety and traditional use in herbal medicine.

Lore is another way we can begin our exploration of any plant person. When we adventure with our favorite ancient heroes or read tales of the old gods, which plants make an appearance? Are they associated with any special feats, blessings, narratives, or deities? How could these associations give us insight into the ways our ancestors related to them? When you look, it's amazing how often plants make an appearance in our greatest tales—I believe they have been added to both invoke their power into the story and as a means to preserve our ancestral connection to them.

We're fortunate these days to have access to a plethora of *materia medica*; books detailing the medicinal virtues of the plants. Almost all traditions of herbalism have these books in one form or another, and websites can even be found that give detailed monographs of a variety of herbs. Having a good materia medica to turn to when researching plants is crucial. They help us learn about the traditional ways the herbs

MEDICINE, MAGIC, AND MYSTERY   171

have been worked with, give insights into botany and phytochemistry, and some even share folklore about the plants. Before investing in one (or several, as tends to be the case), make sure what you're buying and reading is worth your investment. Avoid books that treat plants as tools to be used, presents them in reductionist 'this herb is good for this issue' ways, or speaks about them being 'put here for human use'. I also like to warn students about books that fetishize exotic or threatened plants or those that are part of closed indigenous practices like Palo Santo, White Sage Sweetgrass, Ayahuasca, Blue Lotus, Dragon's Blood, and so forth. In other words, make sure the books you buy are written with the spirit of the plant in mind and are presented with eco-affirming attitudes and a sensitivity to harvesting and preservation.

We also have access to many *materia magica*; books written extolling the magical, spellcraft, and charm virtues of the plants. Unfortunately, most all of these books are presented in a reductionist, allopathic, and utilitarian way instead of the relationship-based way we're really looking for. If you find good books in this genre, make sure to research the plants beyond what's on the pages. Look up photos of the plant, learn the medicinal properties the plant holds, and see if you can find folklore associated with them. All of this should line up- as you learn more about the other aspects of the plant's being the magical virtues should resonate. I'll share some of my favorite books with you in the resources section.

Because our modern world has placed a greater value on the medicinal benefits of the plants than the magical, when they are in fact one in the same if we just look at them from a fuller perspective, it's easier to find information about the healing virtues than the transformative ones. The good news is that with even a cursory understanding of a plant's medicinal virtues, we can explore their magical mysteries.

Examples of this include looking at herbs with an affinity for the cardiovascular system for our workings in love and connections, adaptogens and nervines for cultivating peace, nootropics for intuition and mindfulness, integumentary herbs for protection and boundaries, and herbs aligned to a healthy digestive system for letting go of what doesn't work for us. Blood cleansers and lymphatic herbs can be worked with in purification and cleansing magic, and herbs that bring nourishment and vitality can be connected to for abundance and wealth work. In this way, we meditate on the connections between organs, systems, and processes within the body, recognize them as part of nature, and see how they may reflect to other aspects of our life journey. With this perspective, a top-notch materia medica or monograph can be used as an entry point to learn about the deeper mysteries of any plant. From there, we can approach them with confidence and connection as we nourish a direct relationship to them in journey and ritual.

PLANT SPIRIT MAGIC

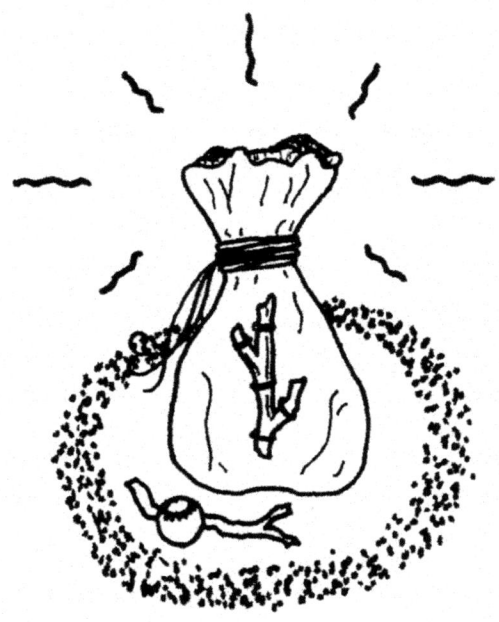

Magic is the arte of creating change from the subtle realms to the here-and-now. Through it, we can transform ourselves and our narratives to better suit who and how we wish to be. Magic is completely natural, fully compliant with the laws of nature, and ultimately an inherent skill within the human being that can be awakened and refined with practice.

Our approach to magic centers the plant spirits as our guides and allies in the work. Where many traditions focus on using the magician's own energy to create change, we ally ourselves to the beings of the green realm to aid us in crafting our transformations. We practice a *relationship-based* form of simple folk magic that connects our will and power to the power and influence of the plant spirits through relationship, ritual, and reciprocity. This is true sorcery in action.

Earlier on, we explored petitions and how we can reach out to the plant spirits to help us when we need their specialized kind of perspective and guidance. Here, we build upon what we learned there and step into more sorcerous acts whereby our world is linked to theirs in making magic. Petitions are essentially requests, prayers even. They are a way for us to take the need from within and express it to those who have the power to respond. Petitions are always magical in their own right, but when combined with ritual actions that ground out the transference of power into our narrative, they become even more so.

There are two key steps to the style of plant spirit magic I work and teach. The first is petitionary, where we approach a specific spirit or group of spirits to ask their help and gain their allyship for our magical workings. The second is to provide a place for their powers to take root in our lives. The petition usually happens in the form of the invocation ritual we've already learned and may include forms of divination to help us clarify the spirit's response. I'll show you some fantastic forms of plant spirit divination later. The rooted aspect of the magic takes the form of incense, sachets, baths, teas, amulets, candles, oils, powders, or other expressions that involve the physical body of the plant spirit we're working with. By this method we approach both *spirit* and *form* to craft truly holistic magic. Just as our goals influence the inner and outer, subtle and dense, passive and active, light and dark part of self, our magic should reflect the same.

As you may have guessed, plant spirit magic is deeply invested in the power of the plants themselves. We are relying quite heavily on them showing up and lending us their virtues. Without their participation, we can still experience quite amazing things happening, but nothing compared to what happens when the plants actively engage. So, much of this work is about making connections, offerings, and journeys dedicated to the plants we seek help from. After that, the power flows easily into our amulets, charms, bags, and blends. I like to think of plant spirit magic in the form of *the three R's*: relationship, reciprocity, and ritual. Just these three things taken into proper consideration and enacted well will result in magical manifestations.

In the previous chapter we learned ways to discover the mysterious virtues of our plant allies. We do this so that we know which plants to call upon when we need aid in specific areas of life; magical and medicinal. We can also turn to the lore, old herbals, and the plants that start showing up in our life at the same time a transformation is needed. When we discover a plant or group of plants that has a special influence or interest in the area of life we are working on, we can approach them through journey or invocation to see if they're willing to help. We communicate with them, share our needs with them, and follow their lead as we step into the journey of magic.

Making magic

Before we begin, let me clear something up. Chances are you're expecting this to get really complicated, have many steps, and be full of pomp. The fact is that folk magic, especially of the animist variety we practice, is deceptively simple. The simplicity of our magical actions makes room for the plant spirits to do what they do best. We are not casting layered circles, raising energies with theatrical gestures, reciting complex litanies, or trying to pronounce languages we've never before encountered. Animistic folk magic relies on the power of connection, allyship, and sincerity. So, don't make the mistake of overlooking what's really possible here—and what really happens when you work good magic.

Our magical workings are a combination of arte and craft. We make a personal connection to the green realm through our arte of journey and dedication and craft a way for virtues to flow and root into our lives. That is all. It's very simple, very intuitive, and very adaptable—as it should be. Your working of plant spirit magic should be informed first and foremost by your own relationships with the plant spirits themselves. To help get you started, here's a framework, the full ritual for most of my plant spirit magics, which you can use as-is or change to suit your own ways.

- Consider your magical goal and explore the plant spirit that might be the best ally for the work. Connect with them in journey, dream, divination, or direct communication to make sure they're aligned to you and your magic and are willing to help. If for some reason they are not, try asking their guidance in selecting another ally who might be a better fit.
- Decide what type of magical working you'll do based on the goal. Will you burn incense, make a sachet, bathe in an herbal wash, burn an herb-rolled candle, or apply an herbal anointing oil or balm to

your body over a set amount of time? The next section details several options of craft to choose from.
- Gather all items and prepare your ritual space, ideally in alignment with lunar and/or solar tides.
- Open a circle of invocation and set out your offerings to the plant spirit. The working is placed in the center of the circle and after the plant spirit is invoked by our usual method, it is either crafted or simply meditated on to connect it with the magical goal. This process is part an expansion of your will and spirit to encompass the work and part a prayer for the plant spirit to channel their virtue into the working. Here, we truly meet the spirits halfway.
- Experience the magic happening. Use your inner vision, senses and feelings, intuition, or other imaginal faculties to *perceive* the process unfolding.
- When finished, put the magic to work. If you crafted a sachet, bring it into your field. Candle should be lit, incense burned, bath prepared, or whatever else you did. Let the beginning of the magical working be anchored in the invocation ritual.
- Finish the invocation ritual as per usual and carry the magic out into your life.
- As your goals manifest, it is important to pay for them. Ensure that you continually make offerings and express specific gratitude to the plant spirit that aids you. In my own practice I dedicate a beeswax candle to the spirit on my shrine and spend a few minutes every day lighting it, offering incense, and laying other offerings. For plants that are safe for me to take internally, I will also usually take a few drops of a tincture as a way to keep connected to the plant spirit as we work together. Our acts of magic are rarely an event and are almost always a process of shifting, transformation, and an opening of new pathways.

Again, because I cannot stress this enough, the process should be simple, sincere, and filled with the energy of kinship. Our magic is about calling the virtues of the great plant spirits into our lives in specialized, sorcerous ways—this type of folk magic looks to the untrained eye like the simple lighting of a candle, burning of loose botanical incense, or bathing in an herbal wash. To those who know, great stores of power, guidance, and transformation are being given to us and our life paths.

With practice and experience you will feel shifts happen in the green world and in our world.

Also remember that our work is about cultivating and nourishing deep spiritual relationships with the plant spirits. As we do this, they will teach us directly, some of them even becoming our familiars or patron spirits. What we get through the inspiration of our practice is more important than anything found in a book. What is documented here reflects generalizations from my own work, guided by the plants, that work for most folks. Creative license is an important part of this work for without it you are limited to the relationships of the author instead of the limitless power of your own journey with the spirits.

What does your magic look and feel like in your mind's eye, and how can you embody this vision and turn it into ritual?

Expressions of plant spirit magic

There are as many ways to anchor in the virtues of the plant spirits as there are magical goals we might be working on. I'd like to share just a small sampling with you to help inspire you and show you how to put the *craft* into your work.

Sachets

One of my favorite ways to carry the magic of my plant allies with me into the world and to really let the transformations sink into self and path is through sachet work. Whether you're a competent sewer or not, these can be effective and even beautiful works of craft.

Start by choosing fabric and thread colors that feel resonant with your goals or the plant spirit you are working with. You can bundle up loose dried herbs from your plant ally into cloth and tie off the top, or sew the dried herb into felt or canvas for a more polished result.

Sachets can be constructed inside of a ritual or made in advance. I like to craft them in a ritual setting and then place the finished sachet inside my invocation circle to charge and set it working.

Once securely tied up or sewn and charged in ritual, sachets can be carried in your pocket, hung around your neck to rest on your heart, or even tied so that they rest on a specific body part. You can sleep with them on your nightstand or under your pillow or give them rest and replenishment by placing them on your plant spirit altar in your working bowl overnight.

Whenever you do any kind of offering or ritual for the plant spirits, the sachet should be placed on the altar to be fed and celebrated alongside them as an expression of your working ally.

You can carry the sachet for a set amount of time like a lunar cycle, until you've met your goal, or forever. When you no longer have need of it, untie or unthread the fabric to undo the binding magic and return the ingredients to the land, base of a tree, or compost bin. Conversely you can keep the sachet as part of your plant spirit shrine to act as a vessel for that plant's spirit.

Incense and bundles

To smolder or burn herbs is to release the power of the plant spirits into space and time. This is perhaps the most ancient and revered way of plant spirit magic, and it is one that commands the attention of all our senses. After charging the loose herbs or dried bundle in ritual, it can be burned in the moment to carry prayers, purify a space, charge an area with a specific energy, or come into the body via sacred breath.

Two simple ways to work with incense made from a single herb is by loosely powdering them to be placed on hot incense charcoal in an urn or bundling them up while fresh and allowing them to dry into the shape of a burn bundle. That first plume of smoke in a ritual is quite inspiring, and really acts to bring in the virtues of the plant spirits.

For those with a knack, incense can be crafted from pure botanical ingredients and charged to make their casual burning that much more potent.

Always make sure that the herbs you choose to work with in incense are safe for inhaling.

Candles

Candles are a celebrated way to work magic for many reasons. They use the symbol and presence of light to shed wisdom and warmth on a situation, they burn with rhythm allowing magical workings to have a defined ritual length, and they act as powerful ways to focus spirit and mind on magical rites.

My favorite way to craft magical herb candles is to finely powder the herb, warm or melt the outer layer of the candle's wax, then roll the candle in the powdered herbs. You can do this several times to really get a nice coating of herb material in the wax. Those who know how to make candles can also add the powdered herbs into a mold or into the wax during dipping.

The candle can be placed in the circle during invocation and lit or charged to be lit later on. Candles can be allowed to burn all at once or lit for some time each day to fire up the magic. I usually keep them on my shrine and set them over a piece of paper on which is written something that links to my goal, usually a drawing.

Be mindful that some candles will burn brighter and bigger with the extra organic material the flame can latch onto. They should be burned on a large heat-proof plate or surface to ensure the fire stays where it's safe.

You can also craft petitionary candles for specific plant spirits, deities, or ancestors in this same way. It's a simple method that adds something really special to the candles we burn on our altars. Anything we can do to bring the plant spirits into our work in deeper ways is always a good thing!

Baths and washes

Cleanse away, wash in, charge walls and floors, or just start fresh. Baths and washes are a lovely way to call in the virtues of the plant spirits and quite literally bathe in them!

Bath and wash blends can be charged in ritual within the bowl, then used later. For a bath, a super strong tea can be made and then poured into a full tub of water, or herbs can be bundled up in cheesecloth and allowed to steep in the tub. You can also make a jar of tea and pour it over your head outside or rinse specific areas of the body as needed. Always make sure you're working with herbs that are safe for use on the skin.

Washes can be made in a similar way. I like to brew a strong, concentrated tea with the plant and then add that to a bit of wash water. This can be used to wash walls and floors, sidewalks and exteriors. Tea can also be added in smaller amounts to the washer to infuse clothing and other fabrics with magical energy. Be mindful that some herbs will stain certain fabrics.

Powders

Powders allow you to spread the energy of the plants around a space easily and effectively. They can be used to sprinkle over a space before sweeping them out as a cleansing ritual, applied to the body, added to incense or candles, or blown onto doors or walkways where a plant's energies are needed. Powders, due to their fine nature, can be irritating to lungs, eyes, and skin- so be mindful if you choose this format of magic.

I like to grind powders by hand in a mortar and pestle set inside an invocation circle. You could also do this in advance using a coffee or spice grinder.

Store powders in a clean, dry glass container and keep away from light, heat, and moisture. Once powdered, the plant materials increase their surface area many times and will break down in color, aroma, and vibrancy very quickly.

Amulets

An amulet is a plant part that is worked with directly. Instead of sewing, burning, or carving, we simply work with the plant material itself. Dried roots, berries, nuts, bark, twigs, or other relatively tough materials can be used. Amulets can be strung on a thread and worn around the neck, carried in the pocket, placed in a pattern around the base of a candle, hung above or on doorways, tucked into glove boxes, or set up at the corners of an area of land.

Amulets have a special affinity for the green arte practitioner, as they carry the signature of the plant very directly. They are, in essence, an expression of magic given from the plant spirit themselves.

Once the magical working has been completed, amulets can be placed on a plant spirit shrine to continue working with the spirt involved or returned to the land. If possible, burying them at the base of the living plant from which they were harvested is an ideal return of power.

Growing

If you have the space and the know-how, growing a plant you wish to work with in a magical context can be a powerful experience. Stewarding a plant in this way is a commitment that shouldn't be taken lightly.

You are inviting them to show up where you are and are promising to care for them for as long as they remain present in your life. I like to do this kind of work for deep workings such as spiritual growth, connection to the green realm, or peace.

My favorite way to do this is to charge both seed or sprout and a small piece of cotton paper with my magical goal written out in some way together in a circle. Then, within ritual, the seed or sprout are planted with the paper underneath them. As they grow, they draw on the magical working and help to bring it into the world with the virtues they channel in naturally.

If the plant is an annual, at harvest they can be worked with to make medicines, incense, amulets, or other magics related to the original goal. If they are perennial, the working should be one that you'd like to invest energy into year after year.

Oils and balms

Applying the energies of the plants to pulse points, the heart center, ailing body parts, candles, doorways, or ritual tools is a wonderful way to anchor their power into our world. Oils and balms are both ancient and celebrated ways of working plant spirit magic, and the intimacy of applying them directly to our skin is a great way to connect more deeply to our green allies.

I like to craft oils and balms for magical workings that I return to time and time again. Balms for spirit flight, protection, and peace; oils for healing, intuition, and divination. Consider this method of magic as one that you craft once and can draw on over and over again until a new batch needs to be made.

You'll find recipes for herbal oils and balms in the grammar.

Tinctures

Bring the magic inside! Tinctures are a powerful way to make both herbal magic and medicine; and ideally a little bit of both. Tinctures let us call the plant spirits past the hedge of our own being and into the depths of who we are deep inside. This is magic from within, and is best suited for those workings that focus on changing our minds, hearts, and bodies for the better. I think that all herbal medicines should be crafted as if they were magical workings. Why not? Adding that extra connection to the spirit or spirits involved in the formula just adds another dimension to the medicine.

Tinctures are forever. Once made properly, they expire when alcohol does—never! In addition to taking them internally in drop or therapeutic doses, they can also be used to anoint the body, candles, sachets, or jewelry and added to baths, washes, teas, and diffusers.

As always, make sure that any tinctures you take are safe for you. You'll find a tincture how-to in the grammar.

Potions

Potions are a concentrated and lightly preserved way to ingest herbal infusions. They're basically tea with a bit more kick and some extra sweetness. Potions are intended to be taken in small doses for a short amount of time as they do have a shelf life. I like to make my potions in the form of an oxymel, which uses apple cider vinegar and local honey as its base.

Potions are a wonderful choice for healing, magics of transformation, initiations, and pre-ritual shots to help ease us into a more spiritual mindset. I like to store mine in small glass bottles that can be easily carried into rituals, taken before a journey, or given to a client to take before a supportive meditation.

When charging your positions, consider the blessings of the Bees and of the Apple spirit as well. They are both potent allies in magic and medicine and make a special appearance here. Pouring a libation for them during the invocation is wise.

Only herbs that are safe to take internally should be worked with for potions. My method for crafting vinegar and honey potions can be found in the grammar.

THE SHARED MEAL

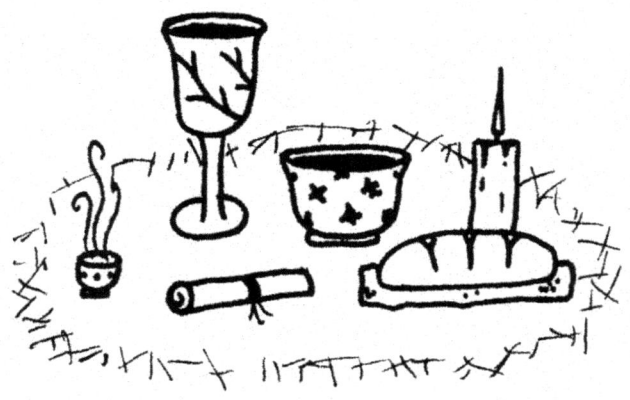

Much of our work is about entering into deeper and deeper states of connection with the kindred, and there are few rituals that accomplish this more powerfully than the shared meal. Throughout almost all of the world's spiritual traditions, animist and otherwise, we see actions of breaking bread, pouring libations, or receiving sacrament. By sharing in nourishment with *other*, we connect ourselves to them and them to us through the medium of sustenance.

For me, the shared meal is a simple ritual of intimacy and power. Through it, we step to meet the spirits halfway and honor the raw personhood of all of us. While the spirits partake in a different aspect of the food than we do, they partake nonetheless. To share a ritual cup and bowl with them is to bring us into rapport and harmony from levels cellular to spiritual.

In the sharing of food and drink, the offering itself acts to bless and fulfill the participants from both sides of the hedge completely. We humans are nourished by the physical substance of the food; macronutrients and the like. Those inhabitants of the spirit world we celebrate with partake of the *essence* of the food; what is known as *foison* in the Scottish ways. They take on the vital force of the food while we take on the substantial force. The intimacy is shown by how one gift, let's say bread and wine for example, can act as a liminal point of connection between two worlds. There's no wonder why the converting religions maintained this sharing of a sacred meal as they absorbed older Pagan traditions.

On a deeper level, the shared meal is a mystery embodied. It is a recreation and an active participation in sacred cycles of reciprocity that fuel the existence of life itself. Through the shared meal we step into a dynamic dance of gift and receipt, host and guest, send out and bring in. This whole process, in ways both subtle and profound, connect us to the cycles of life.

There are two ways to offer a shared meal; one informal and the other part of a larger ritual or fête. We'll cover the informal version in this chapter, and the more involved version in the next. You'll recognize much of this from our earlier exploration of the *full moon rite*. Here, we go a bit deeper into the process, which both builds on that ritual while helping us go further into the work next time around.

What you'll need for the shared meal

- A ritual cup and bowl as outlined in the chapter on *Tools of the Arte*.
- A drink for the cup. Wine, dark beer, dark liquor, herbal tea, fruit juice, or wild waters are all appropriate here.
- Food for the bowl; bread, cookies, pastry, or other foods that have in some way been crafted by human hands are all appropriate. There is power in what we can make—and so our offerings should always include the signature of our work.
- An optional offering bowl into which you can pour libation and set food offerings. If you're outside, this can be done directly onto the land, ideally at the base of a good tree.

And that's all it takes. Keep it simple so that there's plenty of room for the mysteries to unfold. In these quiet, devotional moments we can receive volumes of the mysteries like flashes of lightning or softly uttered poems.

With the above items on the ready, we can work a lovely, shared meal with the kindred spirits. Again, focus on the feeling and the vibrancy of the ritual and keep everything else as simple and clutter-free as possible, so that things flow easily and beautifully.

To enact your shared meal, portions are offered *first* to the spirits and then we take some for ourselves. Many traditions reverse this order and have the individual drink and eat then offer the remainder to the spirits. To me, sacred hospitality invites us to serve our guests first and honor their presence.

Begin with a short and heartfelt invitation to the spirits, like the sample version below. With each verse some of the drink is poured into the offering bowl or onto the ground, making sure that you end up with enough for yourself at the end. You do not have to share meal with all the spirits all the time. This is a lovely rite to honor someone specific.

> *I stand here in the presence of the elder deities, spirits of the green realm, and my good ancestors. In honor of you I share this meal. Please receive these gifts with my love—may they strengthen our bonds of kinship.*
>
> *To the elder deities of our ways: Lord of Leaves and keeper of the gates, great Green Man. Sovereign lady, Goddess of the Land, giver of life and death. I pour this drink for you and ask that you accept it.*
>
> *To the spirits of the green realm: Great plant spirits who are rooted in the otherworld and fruit in this world, givers of medicine and magic, allies in healing and harmony, I pour this drink for you and ask that you accept it.*
>
> *To my ancestors of blood, land, and tradition: Great ones who have gone before me, you who have well-worn the path and left it lit and clear for me, I pour this drink for you and ask that you accept it.*
>
> *In honor and celebration of our kinship, I drink with you! (drink the remainder)*

Now, a bit of the food offering is placed into the bowl or onto the land with the recitation of each verse, making sure to leave an abundant bite for yourself at the end.

To the elder deities: Lord of leaves and keeper of the gates, great green man. Sovereign lady, goddess of the land, giver of life and death. I lay this food for you and ask that you accept it.

To the spirits of the green realm: Great plant spirits who are rooted in the otherworld and fruit in this world, givers of medicine and magic, allies in healing and harmony, I lay this food for you and ask that you accept it.

To my ancestors of blood, land, and tradition: Great ones who have gone before me, you who have well-worn the path and left it lit and clear for me, I lay this food for you and ask that you accept it.

In honor and celebration of our kinship, I eat with you! (eat the remainder)

Thus ends the simple shared meal. This can be done daily, at the bright moon when the spirits are more perceptible in our realm, as part of weekly devotions, or to begin or end any ritual. You can easily work this into any invocations, magical workings, journeys, or even garden chores you may do. There is always cause for celebration in our work, and the more we become attuned to the plant spirits and other inhabitants of the green realm, the more powerful our path becomes.

Celebrate

Find some time, today is the best day, to share a simple meal with specific spirits you've started connecting to or to the kindred in general. Don't overthink it or get in your own way. Show up with an open mind and heart, gifts of love, and an excitement to participate in the obscurities of the green realm.

THE GREEN RITUAL

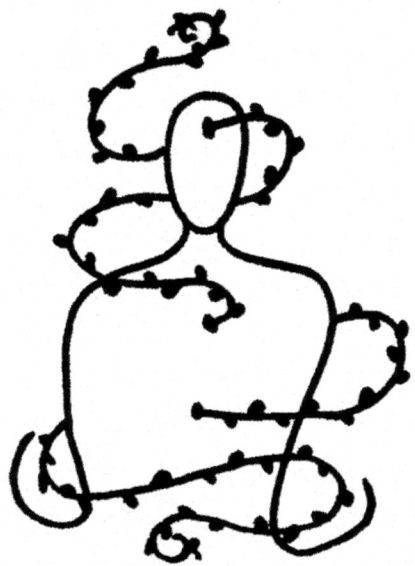

What follows is a ritual framework you can use to support your magical workings, medicine makings, journeys, meditations, seasonal fêtes, or any other adventure into the green realm you choose to take. This ritual flow is intended to be loose to ensure you have plenty of space to make it your own. I follow it roughly as it's presented here because I'm a fan of organic simplicity and intuitive ease, but you should feel free to add or adjust as you feel inclined or are guided by your allies.

When we open a formal ritual space like this, we are stepping into a sacred grove, no matter where we may be. In a backyard, forest, or desert, or in your own living room, the creation of sacred, intentional space acts to transform the ordinary into the liminal. As you do the steps, make room for yourself to slow down or even stop completely so that you can *experience* what is happening. Challenge and test your process to make sure it's as good as it needs to be and stay open to make changes as you grow.

The steps of this ritual flow are:

- Marking
- Cleansing
- Raising the Hedge
- Invocations
- Offerings
- Workings
- Shared Meal
- Devocation
- Releasing the Grove

Let's look at each step in detail:

Marking

To prepare for our rituals, we start by petitioning the spirits of place, marking the space we'll need, kindling a fire, and making an offering. This helps to ensure that we honor the beings who call this place forever home, while we inhabit it for only a short time. It also brings us into closer relationship with the land and the beings who dwell there so that our rituals can go more smoothly and be backed with greater power. Over time, rituals done in the same place can often lead us into allyships with local spirits, which is something very special in our work.

To mark the space, whether in your own living room or somewhere outdoors, walk in a clockwise circle to define how much area you'll need. Play with this a bit until you're sure you have enough room, then pace three times with intention. This is the space you are assuming responsibility for during your rite so hold that in heart and mind as you define the circle and make your paces.

You may wish to recite something for the spirits of place, such as:

> *To all the spirits of this place, spirits seen and unseen, spirits known and unknown, spirits formed and formless, spirits named and nameless, I come*

here to work my arte, and ask your permission and blessing to hold this space. I vow to honor what you share with me and do my best to leave no ill traces of my presence. I ask in these moments for a sign from you if I am welcome ...

After reciting your petition to the spirits of place, take the omen via divination or just by listening from your whole being for a sign, then pace your circle thrice with intention and power. Know that with this pacing you are assuming complete responsibility for the area and all that happens there. You are stepping up as sovereign and steward. The sentiments should be those of a guardian, protector, ally, and beloved. A specific form of divination for exploring permissions of space can be found in the next chapter.

Step to the center of the space and light a candle or small pot fire. In ancient times, space was considered occupied once the hearth fire was lit, so we take inspiration from this tradition and use it in our ritual circles. Once the flame is lit, spend a few moments allowing your spirit to swell and fill the area in the same way the fire fills the space with light. Be aware of the light filling the space and the connection between flame and space.

Finally, make an offering to the spirits of place. A small pinch from your offering tin, a libation, or some other gift can be set just outside the perimeter of your circle as a sign of peace, plenty, and reciprocity, as well as a request for forgiveness of any trespasses or offenses made.

Remember that you are *officially under contract* for this space until your rite has ended. Treat it and all its inhabitants with the utmost respect and be mindful of what you do, say, and embody.

Cleansing

Once we've set up house, so to say, we should clean it. Cleansing is both a physical and an energetic working; one that addresses any clutter that might get in the way of our ritual flow. My preference for cleansing a space is by smoldering purifying herbs while pacing the circle and visualizing the area saturated in a vibrant green cleansing mist. You'll find a how-to and recipe for cleansing burn bundles in the grammar at the end of this book.

If you prefer not to use burning herbs, water, bell, drum, rattle, hydrosol, song, or herbal powder could all make fantastic alternatives.

Raise the hedge

In many magical traditions, a hard-and-fast circle is cast, which keeps energies in and entities out. In the green arte, we honor the perimeter of our ritual space by raising a hedge as explored in an earlier chapter. We surround ourselves through inner vision with ancient trees or shrubs who act to guard the space, filter the movement of energies and beings across the perimeter, and generate a sense of security and connection for those within its bounds.

Another consideration of safety and protection that you might like to explore is the fact then when we are in the presence of the world tree in ritual or journey, whether visionary or symbolic, we are held between an immense canopy and system of roots. I like to experience the protection in this space as if I am held in a great green sphere of vitality. The canopy above watches over me, shelters my work, and protects me. The roots that weave and wind below me create a strong foundation of safety and stability.

Invocations and offerings

You are now in fully liminal, fully sacred space and hopefully you can feel it! It's time to make invocations for any spirits you'll be working with. If you like, you can do a general invocation for all your kindred; deities, spirits of the green realm, and ancestors, or you can focus the ritual on the person or persons you are working with. While this explanation focuses on working with a plant spirit, you can follow the same general outline to invoke a deity or other spirit you have a connection to.

Refer back to the chapter on *Invoking the Plant Spirits* for inspiration.

Working

This space is carved out for anything you want to accomplish in ritual. You may be doing a divination, journeywork or spirit flight, magical working, making medicine, initiation, or communication with a plant spirit. This is also the section where you can perform any seasonal fête celebration or honoring of the seasonal changes.

Shared meal

In the previous chapter we learned a simple way to share in sustenance with the spirits of the green realm. At this point in the ritual, you can perform a shared meal to ground out your work and make an additional offering of gratitude to your allies. It also makes for a nice end to a formal ritual flow and helps the energies of the ritual ease down.

Devocation

The circle of invocation can now be undone, and the plant spirit or other spirits invited to the space can be given gratitude for their blessings and bid farewell in peace and plenty.

Release the hedge

Returning to the center of your circle, call back into vision your hedge. Acknowledge the power, and with a heart full of gratitude, let the boundary return back to the green realm through the land. Re-engage with your surroundings as a way to ground and center in the moment.

Thank the spirits of place for sharing their space with you, and return the land to them by extinguishing the candle with intention and power.

DIVINATION

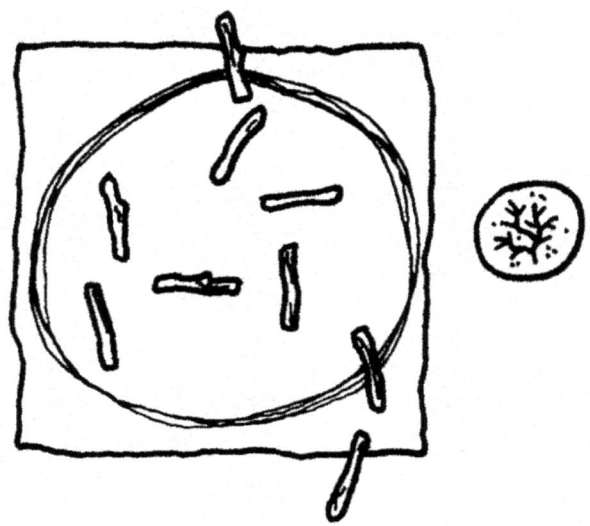

The arte of divination is a more tangible way for us to interface and interact with the world of spirit. Through the various languages of divination, we can ask to be given guidance, permission, or blessings from our allies, all while learning more about the mysterious patterns of nature. In this chapter I'd like to introduce you to several methods of divination used in the green arte. Try them all and see which ones speak most to you. You may find that certain types of divination work best for certain types of spirits or workings and rely on one method for more frequent readings.

Reading the trees

This method of divination can be performed anywhere you have access to tall trees. For me, it is a powerful way to commune with the Green Man, keeper of the verdant gates, but it also works well in communicating with the specific trees involved.

Start by lying on your back under the canopy of a tree or group of trees. Allow your gaze to soften, and explore the patterns made by the leaves and branches contrasted with the sky, sunlight, or moonlight shining through them. Let the movement and sound of the world around you lull you into a light trance.

Within your heart, call up a query. Ask what you need guidance on in a clear and concise way. Be honest and direct. Then, move back into your exploration of the treetop patterns. Soon, an image will emerge that speaks to your query, or you may have inspiration from within gifted by the trees which speaks to your need.

As with all work done in the green realm, make sure you honor what is given as long as it is safe for you. If you receive guidance and ignore it, that guidance will be harder earned in the future.

Casting staves

Working with the wood of a tree ally, you can craft small two-inch or three-inch staves to use as a powerful divination tool. I use a set of nine, a sacred number in the green arte and many animist traditions, but feel free to use as many as makes sense for you. The staves are prayed over for guidance and then dropped or gently tossed. The resulting pattern is read and interpreted.

It is best if the wood for your divination staves is collected by you with proper observances and offerings. Most wood will need to be stripped of bark, sanded, and oiled, which gets you closer to the plant spirit along the way. A bit of your blood can be added to the oil or balm to connect you to the tool. I have a recipe in the grammar for wood wand balm, which works perfectly for finishing your divination staves.

Nature's reply

This method is always with you wherever you go and so it makes for a wonderful way to stay in communication with nature. Inspired by Fionn's Window of the Irish Ogham tradition and Cledonism of the ancient Greeks, it leans into our innate connection with the world and relies on nature's response to give us guidance.

My favorite way to work this divination is to formulate and ask my question at my home shrine. I keep it in mind as I put on my shoes, grab my wallet and keys, and head out the door. From there, I listen for the world to answer what it is I'm seeking in a way that really speaks to the issue at hand. Another way to do this, which is truer to the cledonism technique, is to state your query to your patron deity before entering a busy area like a grocery store or marketplace. It was tradition to plug one's ears until they were in the thick of the crowd, then unplug them and take as advice the first clear thing heard.

With this method it is crucial that we listen for a response that makes sense. I also encourage you not to limit the response to human voices. Animals, car alarms, gusts of wind, smells wafting through the air, and scenes in your field of vision are all equally relevant.

Bones of the land

When working outdoors, getting permission and blessings from the local land spirits is crucial to successful rituals and observations. One of my favorite ways to do this is to find a good palm-sized stone around where I'll be doing ritual, harvesting, plant communications, or even just sitting for meditation. Ask for permission or guidance from the land and be fully attuned to the sensation of the stone in your hand. If the stone lightens as a response to your query, the answer is interpreted as positive, if the stone becomes heavy, the answer is interpreted as a negative.

Replace the stone where you found it and follow the guidance of the land.

Whispers in the wind

The winds are a power recognized in all animist traditions. They are invisible, being known only by their influence on the environment as they gust through. When the winds rustle through trees, they whisper many curiousities—communing as they do with the spirits of place.

This method of divination invites you to still and quiet both body and mind, then listen. Listen intently and from everywhere in your being. Listen for words and phrases, songs and rhymes. Also, listen for feelings and emotions, memories and visions. The winds speak in mysterious ways. Like gazing in the treetops, I have found that this type of divination is very well-suited to communing with the elder deities of nature.

Taking omen

Our hearts are always in communion with the world, and it can be said that the world is always responding to our hearts. Taking omens is a way to navigate what I call *the green thread*. To find places in your life where you're in a great deal of harmony and things are really just lining up—then to keep following it, like pulling a thread.

Omens will come to each of us in unique ways. What is meaningful and out of the ordinary to you might be meaningless or commonplace to me. The sight of a specific bird, an uncanny string of events, the howl of a dog, the limb of a tree cracking in the wind, or other messages that hit as important for you are worth listening to. I am not a fan of wandering through life with eyes aimed at the sky waiting for a sign; life happens *here*. But, when something comes into our field of perception that holds importance in our personal set of symbols, then there is good chance a message is being delivered.

Ogham

For those with a bent toward the more formal divination style, Ogham makes for a powerful companion. This ancient Irish marking script has been used to define boundaries and read subtle patterns for a very long time. Ogham is in essence an alphabet of twenty letters, each one with an array of divinatory meanings. Over the ages, animals, locations, trees, plants, colors, and even sounds have been linked to the Ogham letters making a robust and relevant system of exploration. The Ogham letters are often carved onto small staves of wood, then cast onto a mat or drawn at random from a bag before being interpreted by the reader. Being part of Irish traditional Paganism, it is best to go the extra mile and learn Ogham from native Irish teachers. The Irish Pagan School[2] has some incredible Ogham offerings including history, lore, mysteries, and practical applications.

---

[2] www.IrishPaganSchool.com

Once you've gotten a good handle on the traditional staves, I invite you to consider what a bioregional Ogham alphabet would look like where you live. Which trees are represented in Ogham that don't live where you live? What lists of local animals, landmarks, or other personally relevant Ogham lists could you make?

Divination is all about becoming consciously aware that we are *always in communication with the world*. The conversation is always taking place and we are an integral part of it. Divination in the green arte is an invitation and initiation to re-join that conversation with full presence and participation.

TABOOS

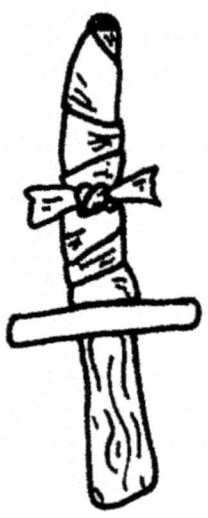

One of my definitions of living an animistic perspective is *just because you can, doesn't mean you should.* Taboos are an important and sacred part of all animist traditions across time and place, and they evolve from the hard-won experience of our ancestors as a way to keep us safe and in honor of right relationships. Taboos are essentially boundaries and unspoken contracts. They help us to know, usually through lore and folktale, what we can and cannot do when we're a guest in the spaces and realms of otherness.

Many Western folks balk at the idea of a taboos because we're neither used to or fond of being told 'no'. We've been systemically conditioned to believe in the toxic notion of human exceptionalism and supremacy, and in micro exceptionalism and supremacies within the human group.

Because we're better, smarter, more advanced, or more chosen, we have fundamental rights to do what we want, where we want, how we want, to whomever we want, with no negative repercussions. This code of anti-ethics goes against the foundational principles of animism and leads us down paths of wanton offence to the spirits. Time and time again I see 'bad things happen to good people' who are working the standard Western model simply because their 'good behavior' in our capitalist society is deeply offensive and worthy of retribution to the other folk who share spaces with us.

So, to work well with the green realm, we must lean into the idea of healthy boundaries, trust in the taboos handed down from our ancestors, and become radically awakened to the fact that the rules in the great sea of spirit are often much different than those on the tiny island of our reality. We must adapt to be excellent guests rather than expecting the spirit world to adapt and let us slide due to our humanity. Those who put the effort in and try hard to be good guests in this work quickly attract the attention of the good spirits and are led further into the mysteries. In fact, if there's one thing any human person can do to begin opening the ways into this work, it's to practice a type of kindness and sensitivity that carries across the hedge and into the realms of other.

While many countless taboos exist in various animist traditions, I have chosen to focus on four that I think encompass many of them. As a student of the lore of your ancestors, you are sure to find more examples, and I encourage you to sit with them all, run them by your allies, and see how they work in practice. For now, let's explore what I consider to be the four most essential taboos in our work.

Don't get in the way

The land is a tapestry of ancient tracks. We see physical manifestations of these tracks in the way wild animals tread lines in the soil and even in the way sunlight and moonlight draw across the surface of the earth. These tracks have existed since time immemorial, and they serve as spiritual pathways by which the spirits can traverse this world and the other. The tracks are powerful because the exist here *and* there. They are dynamic and liminal spaces; crossroads, gateways, bridges, portals, and highways between the realms.

Celtic lore (I use the term *Celtic* loosely throughout this book to honor the similarities and culture-sharing between many related peoples while also recognizing the distinct individuality of cultures commonly given the Celtic label such as Irish, Scottish, British, and Welsh) is saturated with stories from our indigenous animistic traditions of Faery faith about the dangers of blocking or otherwise impeding spirit tracks. Houses built on them, roads paved over them, even naps taken on top of them can lead to great adventures, but more commonly great disasters.

The tracks are part of an unspoken and ancient contract between humans and the spirits of place and beyond. They are an active meditation on the fact that just because we can, doesn't mean we should. These beings, the tracks, and even the animals who follow the tracks have been here longer than us; they were *here first*. The sovereignty of space is theirs. We are guests, and it is crucial that we honor the very small spaces the spirits have claimed to the best of our ability.

Another facet to the taboo of not getting in the way concerns behaviors. Some of the things folks do when they're in a wild or sacred space don't necessarily block the space, but do leave a negative impact on it. Trash, fire debris, tree ties, types of offerings left behind, damage to the soil through trampling, moving rocks around, and the like all count as getting in the way. Our presence in any wild, sacred, or outdoor space should ultimately be imperceptible once we've left, with the exception of any eco-supportive offerings that may remain once we're gone.

Calling by name

One of the most honored of all the traditional taboos relates to the otherworldly folk that we generally know as the Faery. It is understood that to speak their name directly acts as a subtle type of invocation, which can be problematic for two reasons. First, if we call them because we said their name in casual conversation and they show up and there's no party—we've invited guests to a cold fire and empty home, which is a direct offense. Secondly, whatever our frame of mind or the surrounding conversation is when their name is invoked may be offensive to them. Remember that their job is not to make excuses for us. They are hidden folk, and so we must actively seek them out to enter into relationship with them. If we do so and are not careful to observe their ways and our ancestral taboos as much as possible, we might be in trouble. If you go looking for otherworldly connections, know that it is your job to play by their rules.

To honor the taboo, we speak around the direct name of these otherworldly beings, always in the positive, occasionally with a bit of sincere flattery. We call them the good folk, the neighbors, the gentry, the others, the kind ones, the people of peace, the fair folk, the spirits of place, land spirits, and the good spirits all.

Hard metals

We see time and time again in the lore that hard, especially ferrous metals, are taboo in the presence of the spirits. There are countless explanations for this that include iron being harmful to the etheric bodies of the good folk, forged hard metals being too warlike for peaceful spirits, hard metals being a reminder of the human destruction of land and environment, or other hidden reasonings about iron and other hard metals within the ways of the spirits.

In my work, I only use metal tools that are considered soft, specifically those that are prone to *verdigris*—the greening patina of copper-containing metals with age and exposure. Brass, bronze, and copper are about the extent of my metal usage, and I keep these tools away from ritual space, wrapped in dark cloth when not in use. Yes, even my craft and fabric-cutting scissors are wrapped in cloth in a drawer of my working table.

In ritual spaces, feel free to bring in blades crafted from stone, wood, or bone. Anything that needs cutting can be cut with blades that are unsheathed just long enough to make the cut, or they can be cut beforehand.

My harvesting tool is forged from bronze with a hawthorn wood handle. I also have pruning shears that I bring out as needed with the proper sensitivity to the taboos. I usually do this by announcing to the spirits of place that I am about to draw a blade in peace for whatever purpose I am using it for. When finished with the task at hand, I re-sheath or re-wrap the blade and state to the spirits of place that it is now put away.

Food

When visiting the realms of the other folk, it is advised quite strongly and in many countless instances that food not be ingested. If we eat while we're there, we nourish our bodies with substances not of our world, and it draws us into theirs.

This taboo should be understood clearly—food should not be taken with or from the good folk when journeying to their world. Food shared with them *from our world* is just fine. Our shared ritual meal happens here, with our food, and them as our honored guests. In that instance, they are actually partaking of food from our world which does not influence them nor us adversely.

In some traditions, food which has been offered to the dead is no longer suitable for consumption by the living. I agree with this completely. Food left on a shrine for *any* of the spirits as an offering no longer belongs to you and must be returned to the land. Food shared in a ritual meal is different. Each participant's drink and bite is portioned out individually thus creating a clear boundary between what is given and what is received.

Plant taboos

There are many taboos in lore and tradition that focus on the plant spirits specifically. While I don't follow many of these myself, I think it's an interesting study to look at them and contemplate them.

A few of these taboos include:

- Only harvesting plants with bare feet.
- Only harvesting plants by holding them in the right hand and cutting them with the left. Sometimes this is reversed.
- Being naked or dressed in a specific color, often white, when harvesting plants.
- Either walking away from a plant without turning your back to them, or walking away without looking back at them, especially after harvesting.
- There are many references to types of metals appropriate for digging, planting, and harvesting. These often strictly forbid the use of iron.
- Plant cuttings should not be allowed to touch the ground, or their vitality will return to the land.
- Taboos related to the tides are plentiful and vary based on tradition and plant. Some plants are to be harvested or planted only during specific moon cycles, some must be planted or harvested under specific astrological signs or times of day, and many taboos are related to interacting with plants in the daytime or in the dark of night.

As you ally yourself to individual plant spirits and the inhabitants of the green realm in general, you will likely be given taboos as part of that journey. Things that feel fine now in relation to the work will start to have an uncomfortable or challenging feeling, which is an indicator that a taboo may be present. You might also receive direct taboo from a plant spirit, deity, ancestor, or other spirit as part of your work. I consider these taboos to be fully contractual and will go to great lengths to honor them *as long as they make sense*. If a taboo was ever presented to me that didn't align with my ethics, put myself or others in harm's way, or felt otherwise problematic, I wouldn't accept it at face value. These opportunities would be an invitation to get more information, learn the perspective of the others, and possibly even negotiate them.

STEWARDSHIP AND SOVEREIGNTY

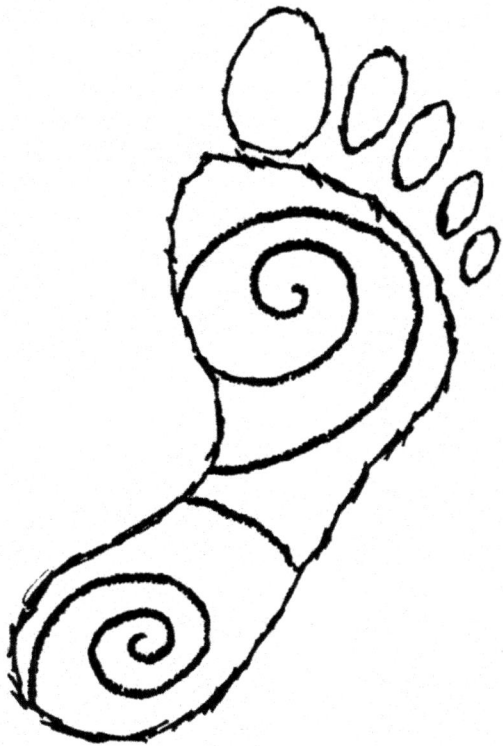

Our work with the plant spirits is a call to engage more intimately with their spiritual reality and also with the physical space they hold in this world. It's all too easy to forget that plants are more than the way we exoticize and fetishize them for our magic and medicine. They have real bodies in time and space, right here in the same world we do. Part of working the green arte is acting to protect and nourish the plants as they grow around us. To defend trees, protect forests, stand up for threatened stands, and even to garden are all ways we engage right here, right now, with the spiritual reality of the plant people.

Where plants grow near you, especially those you have a personal connection to, but all of them really, you have an unspoken contract to honor. The plants who clean the air, feed the animals, break the winds, hold the soil, and catch the rain are all doing you, yes you, a direct blessing. So, if you want to be initiated deeply into the mysteries, step up and take personal responsibility for the community that grows where you grow. The trees and plants in your backyard, in the park down the street, around your place of work, and in your garden are all in your stead. If not yours, then whose?

These plants of your local area are the ones who encounter you every day. They are the ones you run your hands over as you walk by, watch as they enact their yearly life cycles, enjoy as they share their beauty and aroma, and look up in plant books out of curiosity for just who they are. They are your kin, and it is up to you to meet them halfway and be their kin in return.

Simple measures of stewardship go a long way with the spirits of the green realm. Picking up trash, offering water, removing ropes and signs attached to them, applying herbal salves to their wounds, and spending time in communication with them all mean a great deal. If you see them as people, experience them as kin, and treat them as sacred members of your own life you will find that they are given an access to your magic and medicine you never thought possible.

For those who garden, know this to be a sacred work. To invite a plant into your world by seed or by sprout is quite powerful. You are acknowledging a desire to know them in person, to care for them, to watch their life cycle, and to be drawn into their verdant inscrutabilities. When they show up, take it as an act of communication and follow the track.

When it comes time for harvesting, do the right thing. Educate yourself on the best way to cut, prune, and receive from each plant you work with and what time of the season is best for them. Use tools that are held sacred in your work. Speak to the plant, get permission, state your intentions truthfully and candidly; don't beat around the bush! Offer healing balm to the places where branches are cut or trimmed and check on them throughout the year for signs of distress, infection, or disease. Use all of what you take. Take only what you truly need and actively nourish and protect the rest.

The plants, animals, and many spirits of place share space with you. To be truly sovereign, you must step into the role of guardian and servant. We humans are not here to dominate, take, horde, or control. Rather, we have special virtues, areas of influence, and skills, just as the plants do, that put us in a position of great value to them. Our hands can craft and change the state of things. Our minds can link with our hearts to make the imagined a reality. Sovereignty means that our virtues, powers, and privileges are dedicated in as many ways as possible to the land we're on. It is sacred.

Stepping up

Are there places near you where you could step into a stewardship role? Without needing to be a professional arborist or botanist, there are always things we can find to do to be helpful. Is there a park you can dedicate some time each week to picking up trash? How about study time you could do under a nearby tree as a form of communication? Are there trees or plant stands in your area that are threatened? How could you act as a voice for their wellbeing? How are the plants in your own backyard? Is there room for greater connection there?

SHRINE AND GROVE TENDING

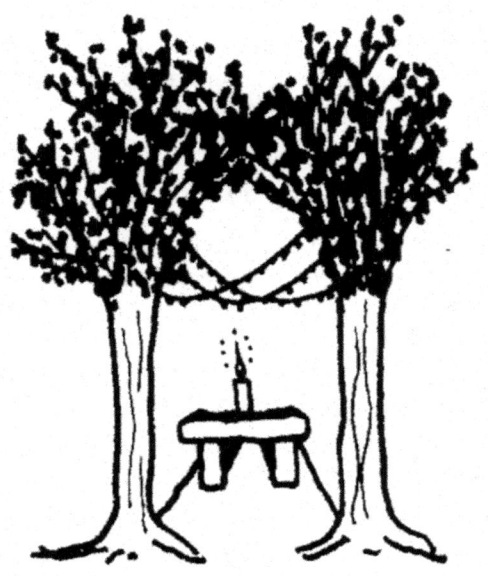

Earlier on we explored the liminal power created when a space is set aside for the presence of the plant spirits, deities, ancestors, and other allies. This space, the shrine, plays a central role in much of our spiritual endeavor and quickly becomes something incredibly exceptional to us. Those of the otherworld who we love and have a great deal of trust and dedication to are represented and invited there, so it is a place filled with magic and medicine. Similarly, those fortunate enough to have access to outdoor spaces where sacred trees, groves, or shrines can be established, often have a deep and abiding love for these sacred grounds.

Tending to sacred space is an evolving act of radical beauty. It changes as we change and reflects the current state of our spiritual journey. As much as the shrine is an offering to the allies, it is also a place to reflect on where we've been, where we are now, and where our journey may be headed.

For those who are new to setting up a shrine or who would like some additional inspiration on how to do so, I offer you these general suggestions to aid in your adventure. I will also share what I consider to be the *bare minimum* tending that should be given to such sacred spaces. As we covered in the chapter on plant spirit vessels, if the spirits are invited and made welcome, they must be attended to. Don't invite them to an empty table!

Setting up shrine

This guidance can be applied, creatively, to both indoor and outdoor shrines. Those in a living room or bedroom corner can be just as powerful as those at the base of an ancient Oak tree or in the middle of a Beech copse.

The shrine should be a space set aside, sacrificed from your own space, for the spirits of your green arte and craft. While only those spirits you're close to or are working with actively should have a space there, it is good to keep a space for each of the three kindred *in general*: the deities, the plant spirits, and the good dead. These three kin form the basis of our allyships in the green arte, and so even if we don't have strong allies in any or all of the groupings, there should be a place of honor for each so they can speak up and speak through.

Your patron deity or deities can be represented in the center of the shrine with statues, photos, symbols, or anything else that works for you and them. In the Green Arte tradition we usually focus our deity devotions to the Green Man or Horned God and the Sovereign Lady, Goddess of Land. The plant spirits can be represented to one side of center individually as explored in that chapter, and a tree statue can be kept as a way to honor *the plant spirits all*. The mighty dead can be represented to the other side of center by a skull intertwined with silk Ivy, photos of your beloved ancestors, family names, or some other appropriate representation.

A green cloth can be laid on the surface of the shrine before the vessels and statues are placed on it. Wood blocks, tree slices, or other items can be used to hold different vessels at good heights.

SHRINE AND GROVE TENDING 211

Along with these core representations, you can also add in other meaningful items, such as icons for animal spirits, land spirits, or other spiritual allies in your arte.

The shrine is now made and will come more alive the more you work with it and the allies who have been offered space on it.

Seasonal reflections

Since honoring the changing seasons is such an important part of staying aligned to the tides of nature, the shrine is a fantastic place to do it. Consider seasonal decorations you can bring in to gather the energy of the seasons and stay attuned to it in your daily workings.

Vases of seasonal flowers, dried berries and nuts, barren twigs, evergreen boughs, dried citrus, herbal blends, garlands, animal bones, color schemes, sacred symbols, and more can all be used to call forth specific virtues in your sacred space.

The tree icon you work with on your shrine can also be decorated seasonally. This is how I align my own shrine to the seasons and it makes for a beautiful offering to the spirits all and a point of powerful contemplation as we circle the year.

Fire

Aside from the representations of the allies, there are a few other things you'll want to keep on your shrine. First and foremost, some way to kindle a flame. This is an offering to the spirits of your shrine, a symbolic lighting of the path, and a recognition of the sacred space your shrine holds.

A beeswax candle (or several) is the perfect way to do this and keeps things nice and simple. I have a small candlestick for the plant spirits and one for my ancestors. The Green Man has two candlesticks which sit on either side of the wooden dais his statue rests on. These candles are lit for pretty much any working or time spent at my shrine. I keep a brass snuffer to avoid having to blow the flames out directly, which is often considered to be somewhat aggressive to the spirit of the flame.

An oil lamp can also be a lovely shrine light but requires more upkeep and a bit more attention to keep things safe as they are known to get out of control if not trimmed and filled properly.

Sacred symbolism

Feel free to add any imagery to your shrine that makes sense to your arte. My own shrine is backed with a carved image of the world tree and is draped with silk Ivy vines and wire lights.

If the deities you work for have special symbols, it's a great idea to include them to make the space more powerful.

Making offerings

The shrine isn't just there to look nice and give us comfort. It is an active, living, and open sacred space where work is to be done. The longer the shrine is tended, the thinner the veil that separates it from the green realm becomes.

The most important thing to do once your shrine is set up is to use it as a liminal place to make offerings. We are given *so much* from our guiding deities, the plant spirits, the spirits of place, and our mighty dead—we often have no real count on the blessings that actually surround us. When we show up ready to give back, we are noticed and responded to quickly. Ultimately, the green arte, like all animistic pathways, is devotional in nature.

Offerings should be made from the heart in ways and with items that are meaningful to you. A special bowl can be kept on your shrine to receive offerings, or you can keep a small bowl at each of the three sections, which is what I do. I also have a small offering bowl outside my back door on an old tree stump which receives offerings to the spirits of place—what goes into this bowl always includes gifts for the tree squirrels who live around my house.

You can add offerings of food, drink, and other gifts in the offering bowls day by day or have one day a week set aside to *feed the spirits*. I do this on Fridays, which we call *Feydey* around my house. Each Friday the offerings of bread, honey, candied fruits, chocolate, and liquor from the week before are removed. The bowls and cups are cleaned and dried, then replaced with new offerings. I will also make offerings during the week which are added to what's already there. If you place an offering that can go bad or might attract fruit flies, leave it overnight and remove it the next day. Offerings of food should be composted or put into a yard waste bin whenever possible. Do not eat, wear, or otherwise use what's been offered. It is no longer yours and would be considered theft. If you have curious animal companions, consider keeping your offerings in glass jar with well-fitting lids.

You may notice that no matter how present your allies may be, the offerings you leave don't vanish. Have no fear, they're not being refused! The spirits partake of the spiritual essence of the gifts, not the physical. They receive the vital force and virtue of the offering leaving the physical form behind. Another reason not to eat what's been offered is that it becomes *negative* in vital force and will often cause sickness when ingested.

Aside from food offered daily or weekly, many other gifts are treasured by the spirits. The most important thing is that the offerings have been crafted by human hands. These don't need to be your human hands, but when you get really close to the allies it becomes more important that it is your virtue they find in what's offered up. Art, incense, oils, tea, sculpture, song, dance, poetry, music, service, décor, and vows are all valid and valuable offerings. Follow the promptings of your allies and green guides and you'll always bring gifts of love that are well received.

If you're stumped on what to offer, consider reading the lore about what the deities of your arte favor. Look at the foods and drinks most valuable to you and give a bit to the spirits. A shot of your morning coffee, a cookie from the pack, or the first tear of a freshly baked loaf of bread are all great gestures. When in doubt, bread and wine are always appropriate—especially if the bread is made by your hands.

Petitions and prayers

The shrine is a powerful place to make petitions and prayers. You can light a candle, set some incense as an offering, and invoke the spirit you're calling out to, asking them to hear your prayer. Keep it simple, honest, and heartfelt and I am confident you will be heard. Take time after prayers to be still and quiet—it is often in these moments that we hear the responses of our allies.

Petitions are more ritualized forms of prayers, and they can take many forms. A written request left on your shrine, an item representing your need hung near a sacred grove, or a song sung in request. Often something is left on the shrine that holds space in the liminal realm for what it is you're after.

I ask my students to wait a full year of entering the green arte before asking for anything other than *a closeness of kinship*. This way, we show up and do the work first with no immediate expectation of getting more from the spirits than they already give. Most folks who come to magical practices are in search of power and wishes granted. To be the exception to that common occurrence makes you stand out to the spirits you call upon.

Taboos

A few taboos are worth noting and reiterating regarding shrine tending:

- What is offered is gone. Do not eat, use, or repurpose what has been given.
- Never keep empty offering bowls on the shrine. There should always be something given- even if that's just fresh water. Bowls and cups can be turned upside down when not in use or kept away in a cupboard.
- Don't use the shrine for anything other than a shrine. This is not a place to set car keys, wallets, or drinks. What is placed on the shrine belongs to the spirits and the green realm. Unless you're not too attached to your wallet and all it represents, keep that somewhere else.
- Avoid offering anything that is not eco-affirming. Consider the long term of whatever you gift. Will it compost? What will you do with it once you want it off the shrine? How will it fare in nature? What will happen if the birds eat it?
- The vessels and statues of the spirits should be honored as being embodied by them. Be mindful of what you do and what you say in front of the shrine as it is heard by the realm of infinite possibilities.
- Care for the physical nature of the shrine. Keep it clean, organized, and beautiful.
- If folks in your life don't respect the arte, keep their hands off your shrine and other sacred items.
- All offerings should have the skill of human hands on them.
- Don't lie to the spirits. Approach them in honesty and forthrightness.
- Be mindful what you ask for.
- Do the work.

Opening vessels for the deities

Should you choose, after some time of consistent dedication, to consecrate a statue of the deities, you can follow the same general outline as explained in the plant spirit vessels chapter. Make adjustments where needed, but the same process works wonderfully for the deities of the green realm.

Once opened, be mindful that a spark of their virtue tends to reside full-time in the vessel. Ensure that they are always well received and that they never go long without your attention and devotions.

WRITING CHARMS, PETITIONS, AND RITUALS

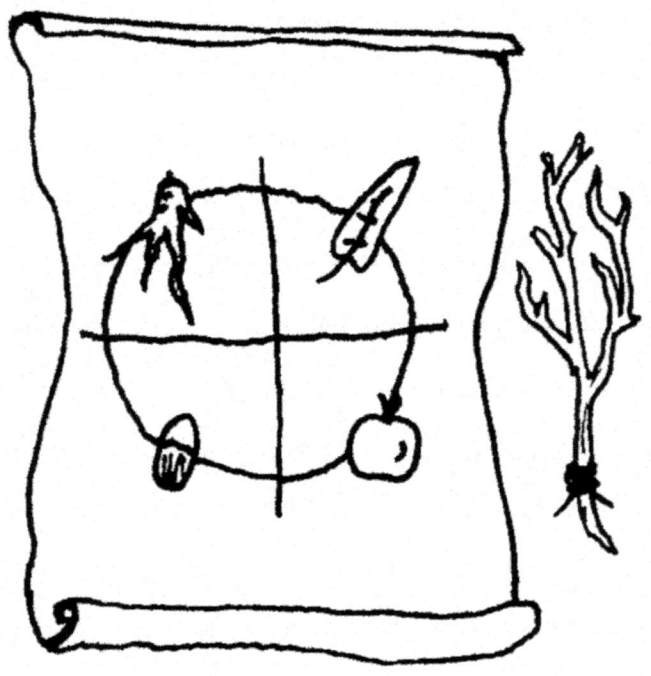

The green arte evolves in the hands of each person who carries it. For this reason, like all nature-based, animistic paths, it stays relevant to the times. Our ability to work with core concepts and tools to craft magic and medicine that speaks to who, when, and where we are is one of the great boons of this arte, and it is an invitation for you to write your own grammar.

Many of us have been conditioned to believe that only old charms are good charms, only recipes from a book are powerful, only petitions recited in an ancient tongue have magic, or that rituals created by us are somehow *less* than the rituals created by someone else. Always remember that sorcery is about relationships, the green arte is about allyships,

218   THE GREEN ARTE

and the way of the green realm is about showing up and doing the work. Charms, petitions, and rituals based on your own experiences with the spirits you are allied to will always carry a beauty, harmony, and potency that cannot be unrivaled by repeating the words of someone else regardless of how imperfect you might think they are.

So, as we move further down these ancient tracks, how do we go about writing good charms, petitions, and rituals? Let's explore.

A charming charm

Charms are words, usually pithy and often rhyming, that can be said once or repeated endlessly to call forth spirits, change consciousness, or align the energies of place. Charms carry a magic all of their own because they focus the will and call forth our virtue - but when combined with the relationships of our arte, they become exceedingly potent.

You can compose a charm to help enter trance, to invoke a close plant spirit ally or deity, to ward off negative energy, or to begin and end a ritual. I suggest beginning by writing out what you really want the charm to say in your own everyday words. From there, you can begin to mold the phrase into something that rhymes, has a nice cadence, or just rolls nicely off the tongue.

Charms are meant to be recited with vigour and confidence, and they should sound beautiful, in my opinion. A simple two-line poem makes a lovely charm that's easy to remember and can build tremendous power.

Here are a few examples of charms you might like to use for inspiration in your own crafting:

A charm to raise the hedge

I pace this circle of sacred ground,
seed to hedge, round and round.
A boundary of green and verdant light,
Protects my body while I take flight.

A charm to invoke the green man

By Oak and Pine,
by Ivy and Vine.

A charm to honor the ancestors

Guardians and Guides from the other side
The mighty dead in green and red.

An act of petition

Petitions are like prayers with the addition of action. They're a way for us to show up fully for our request, and to make a ritual gesture that helps to solidify the process both in our own minds and in the green realm. Taking prayer from something that happens inside the head or on the breath and bringing it out into the world changes it into something quite magical and powerful.

In my petitionary work, I usually state my prayer with the help of a candle offering. I like birthday size beeswax candles for this and will sometimes roll them in powdered herbs or inscribe them with a word or phrase. You can also write down your petition and leave it hanging from a sacred tree or on your shrine, sculpt something that symbolizes your request, or make some other offering that relates to the need.

For those who struggle with more freeform, spontaneous prayer, petitions can also be incredibly helpful. They give us a chance to write out how we're feeling and thinking, and what we're asking for in advance so that we ensure our requests are delivered with clarity. The process of writing out a petition can often lead to guidance from our allies before we've even recited it.

Petitions should be short, sweet, honest, and forthright. Don't beat around the bush and don't sugar coat anything. The spirits don't need you to protect them from your reality. What they do demand is kindness, devotion, sincerity, and gratitude. We have so few opportunities in our lives where we can just show up exactly as we are and be wild and raw in our authenticity. Petitions are a time when all of that is important.

After writing or speaking a good petition, you should have a sense of relief in your heart. You may not feel better completely, but you should feel heard.

If you're new to the petitionary process, I invite you to perform this simple request. Although I suggest waiting some time before asking for things from the spirits, this is an exception.

A petition on the path

To work this petition, you'll need a small candle such as a birthday cake candle or a tealight.

Hold the candle between your palms and against your heart. Just breathe and become present. The wax should begin to warm with the vital force of your body.

Consider your petition and who it is you're asking it of. Imagine infusing the candle with an energy, light, sound, image, scene, or other expression that represents or embodies your request. Once you feel it's been fully charged with your prayer, set it on a shrine or nice surface and light it.

As the flame picks up, invoke the attention of the spirit or deity you are reaching out to and recite the petition. In this moment we are simply asking for guidance on the path of the green arte from the plant spirits all.

Your petition could go something like this:

> *I call out to the mighty plant spirits who are gathered 'round the world tree at the center of the green realm. Great and verdant spirits, givers of magic and medicine, ritual and rightness, beauty and harmony, I ask you to hear my petition which is spoken from my heart to yours ...*
>
> *As I embark on these ancient tracks to wander through the green realm, I ask your guidance, blessings, and inspiration. May those among you who align to my work be made known to me, and may I always be received as a welcome guest in your world.*
>
> *My gratitude and love to the plant spirits all!*

Allow the candle to burn out while you meditate, journal, study, divine messages in the rising smoke of botanical incense, or just enjoy a cup of herbal tea.

Writing rituals of rightness

There are few tasks more daunting to a student of the arte than writing a ritual from scratch. But this process need not be the source of terror. Rituals are poetry in motion, prayer in action, and a recreation of the cycles of the plant spirits. Keeping this in mind, you have creative license to craft rituals that speak to the plant allies you are connected to and the ways you like to align to the seasons and the fêtes of the green ways.

A good ritual follows the tree. It has roots, which represent the real goals of the rite and how it's grounded in reality. The trunk is how we manifest the ritual in its external form—the actions, words, and various trappings that make it sacred. The leaves are our prayers catching the rays of the sun, and the fruits are the successful outcome of whatever is being celebrated.

It is better to enact a ritual with deep roots and a simple exterior than a grandiose and theatrical event with a shallow heart. The simple lighting of a candle, setting of incense, and a heartfelt acknowledgement of the blessings of the season often carry more power than any play-length enactment. I'm a fan of keeping things simple and trying new simple things. I think every year at every season I change things up in one way or another to see how they feel, allow my rituals to change as I grow as a person, and to always make space for the spirits to guide me further down the tracks.

Your rituals should make sense to you and feel good. They may feel *awkward* at times, but overall they should feel *right*. You can use the shared rituals in this book as a guidepost or wander in your own way and make something that fits how you journey. Ultimately, rituals are an offering to the spirits that celebrate their providence and mysteries while helping us align, attune, and grow.

THE KEEP

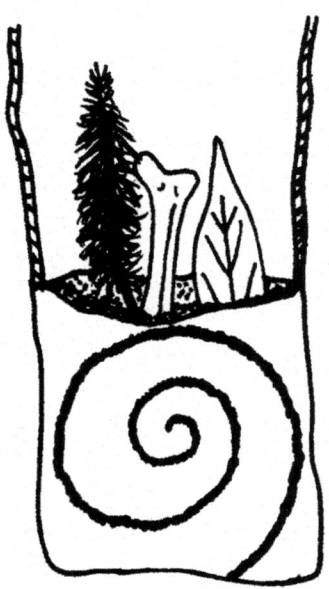

One of my favorite ways to stay attuned to the work I'm doing, and the work being done on me, is to utilize what I call *the keep*. This is essentially a very small sachet, bag, or bundle that is worn around the neck or tucked into the pocket. It acts as a sort of traveling shrine that comes with you wherever you go and keeps you in direct contact with the plant spirits and deities you're closest to. The keep evolves, changes, fills up, empties out, and fills up again endlessly. It is a living mirror of your path and one that acts as a point of liminality and green blessings.

My version of the keep is a small felt sachet, about two inches in diameter, that is stuffed with dried plant materials. Throughout the year I will untie it and change what's inside, refresh some of the materials, or start from scratch as needed. It always contains plants that are sacred to my patron deity, my plant familiar, items related to the season, and bits of my closest plant allies—especially ones I'm more intimately exploring at any given time.

The keep is personal, sacred, and part of you. It should be kept against your skin whenever possible and not shared with anyone else. When not being worn, it should sit on your shrine or hang from a sacred tree to honor what it represents.

I suggest using the *plant spirit invocations* ritual to open your keep and imbue it with vitality and the presence of your allies. You might do this seasonally, once per year on the same date, or whenever the need arises.

The comfort, protection, guidance, and inspiration that comes from dedicating a bit of your personal space to the presence of the green spirits has many far-reaching benefits and can help to greatly deepen your connections and devotions.

THE WILD WITHIN

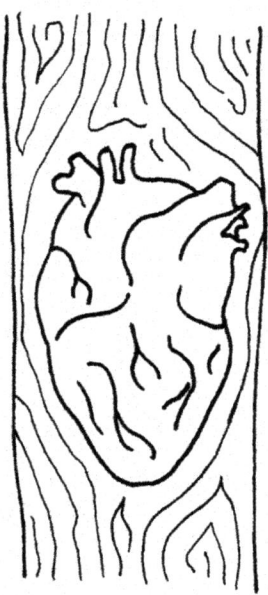

The heart is in constant communication with the whole world.

As an organ, the heart is responsible for pumping nutrients and oxygen to every cell of the body via the vascular system. This means that even more than the musculoskeletal or nervous system, the heart is connected to every part of our being. What is put into the heart is brought to the entirety of the person.

By location, the heart is in the center of the body. Positioned between the brain with all its logic and analysis and the gut with its intuition and instinct, the heart occupies a place that has access to thinking and feeling, embodiment and reaction, remembering and interpreting.

The heart has a beat for as long as the body lives. Each pump of the heart's chambers creates a rush of blood that can be felt as a palpable beat at the pulse points and in the chest. This beat occurs in our world, but in the spaces between the pulses, the heart beats in the world of otherness—in the green realm.

Through and through the heart is our own internal liminal space. It is a crossroads within that connects us to all levels and aspects of our being *and* to all levels and aspects of the natural world. Each of us journeys through life with this living compass beating at our core, acting as a waystation by which the virtues and wisdom of nature can flow to and through us.

To work on the heart is to work on the whole self. As mentioned above, what we put into the heart is pumped to the fullness of who we are. I often guide my students and clients on a drum-driven meditation where they take a drop dose of tincture and allow it to flow into their hearts using their imaginal faculties. From there, the medicine condenses, then expands to saturate all of who they are. This process also guides the individual to find the parts of their being what are blocked, stagnant, or otherwise out of harmony. Where the medicine struggles to flow there is work to be done.

I also like working with forest or garden symbolism within the space of the heart. By coming up with an imaginal wild space, which we can explore using our inner vision, we can come to learn more about who we are, where work is needed, and where the power is. After some time, this space begins to respond to our attention and will work with symbol and feeling to give us guidance from the crossroads. We find that as we visit through journeywork specific plants show up, others change shape or bring messages, feelings change, seasons shift, and the green realm speaks to us through our own hearts. I invite you to work with the meditation below to cultivate, explore, and heal with the symbolism of the wild within.

The wild within

Make yourself comfortable. Working with the green breath, enter into a light trance and connect to the green realm through your inhalation and exhalation.

Place a palm gently on your heart center. Breathe into this space and exhale from it. Activate the heart with openness, expansiveness, and power. Lean into the liminal crossroads that exists within you.

Using your inner faculties of spiritual vision, open a space within your heart and invoke a scene of wildness. Allow the space to show up however it does. Explore this place. See how it feels to be here. Which plants, if any, grow here? What does it smell like? Is the ground bare or covered, soft or dense? Are animals present? Which ones? Do any of the plants or trees in your heart stand out or call to you? Is the space barren and desolate or packed with green beings?

This is a journey of deep personal symbolism. Here you can explore how your heart center appears to you with your own spiritual language. You can also perform great works of healing and magic here. By communicating with the plants of this place, pruning, harvesting, and planting you can add your wild touch to the wild spaces within.

One powerful way to create magic here is to plant a seed in your imaginal wild space. This seed is charged with something you'd like to grow in your own life, and it is nourished and protected by you with both regular visits to your heart space and with actions taken in your usual waking state to cultivate it.

I encourage you to build something in this space—to add your touch. You might create a sacred shrine that represents your spiritual path and links you to any deities you work with. You might create a grotto, platform for sitting, a mirror for reflections, or anything else that feels like what you want and need in this wild place. Adding your touch is adding your own virtues to the place and reaffirming that you are part of nature.

Whenever you desire you can return to this place to explore, learn, relax, create magic, do healing, or just be. The more time you spend here the more you will find the space evolving and responding to you in clear and empowering ways. I like to visit the wild within each night as I drift off to sleep. Here I can review my day, attend to any areas of my inner space that appear dry, malnourished, disconnected, dark, or broken, and fall asleep with healing underway.

If you're doing this work as a meditation, return to your usual state with some gentle massaging, tapping, rocking, and slowly opened eyes.

THE PLANT PRIESTHOOD

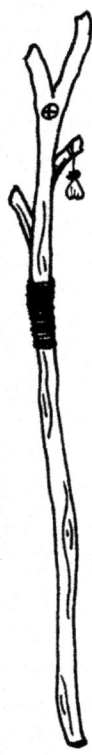

So, what to do with all the wisdom and experience that comes from our work with the plant spirits?

I propose to you, dear reader, a living priesthood of folk who hold the teachings, medicine, and magic of the green realm and work to share it with the world around them. I imagine many of us stepping into roles of guardians, guides, and ritualists for our respective communities and acting as liaison between the world of the plants and the world of humans—for the good of all.

Not all who love the plants will feel called into work on the level of priesthood, and not all who desire it will attain the subtle and epic initiations that accompany the journey, but there is a place for all of us.

From gardeners and foragers to forest protectors and seed keepers. We are, each and every one of us, intimately wrapped up in the way of the plants, and to embrace this fully and with our whole-hearted intention is an act of harmony unto itself. However you feel called and inspired, I sincerely hope you follow.

One aspect of a living plant priesthood that I often dream about is the establishment (or rather re-establishment) of sacred groves and sacred trees, which are of a public or semi-public appreciation. In these spaces we can come together to honor the changing of the seasons, celebrate the old deities, sit in quiet reflection, dance in circles, or journey alone or with others into the green realm. Sacred trees and groves have been a crucial part of our animistic and pagan roots since time immemorial—and I think it's high time we invite them back.

Imagine the effects on all forests, all plants, all trees when they regain their position as sacred symbols and sacred presences. It becomes quite difficult for us to dishonor contracts, ignore taboos, or act in destructive ways when we become aware that the green ones are the provenance of our spiritual wellness, medicines, magics, and sustenance.

Those who are able to establish tree shrines or sacred groves can step into position as priest of those liminal spaces where healing and harmony happen. They may be in your own backyard, a public park, or an ancient forest. No pomp and circumstance are needed here. Just as our home shrines become places of great power after years of work, so too these trees become places where can more easily access the other realms. They might *look* ordinary to the uninitiated, or they may be surrounded with the many trappings of our work, but either way the gateway is open and the magic and medicine flow freely. Around these groves, small groups of herbwise folk can come together as a working *copse* group to honor festivals, enact rituals, learn, share, and steward.

As priests of the plants, *priests* being used as a gender non-specific title, we're invited into a deep bioregional relationship with the way nature shows up where and when we are. We can certainly learn about and explore the plants from other parts of the world, but those who share the land with us have an immediately sacred affinity with our work. Knowing them, we can steward for them, work with them in ritual, cultivate them for magic and medicine where appropriate, and introduce other humans to them. That last point, the introduction, is as close as we might come to proselytization! I have found time after countless time that when human folk learn about the personhood of some local tree, herb, or weed and get lore, stories, virtues, traditional uses, and so forth—something happens. The animism that lies dormant in their blood and bones begins to stir before our very eyes.

We can also cultivate specialized forms of divination that can be worked in service of ourselves and our communities. The trees who grow near us can be worked with to make a bioregional tree oracle inspired by the Ogham of Irish traditions. Certain plants can be worked with in symbol to craft divination systems, or we can simply define good places to go and listen to the trees whisper their secrets.

Where medicine is concerned, there is a special kind of healing that happens when the plants that become our teas, tinctures, salves, and steams grew with the nourishment of the same land that cares for us. We are already in harmony, in relation, so the medicine feels more familiar and goes in a lot deeper. These are the plants we get to watch wake up in the spring, bloom as the summer comes, flower and fruit, then release into harvest. We know them because they make up the world we call home.

Magically speaking, working with the plants of our unique locale invites us to learn the virtues of many plants without the support of traditional lore or monographs, since we might not live in the same place where those stories were told. We are required to sit with the plants of place, observe them, talk with them, and dream about them. We might find ourselves reaching out to local universities, botany groups, plant ID apps, or foraging books to learn more about who shares space with us and how we can enter into deeper relationships with them. Our magics begin to follow the pace of the plant people—we work with who grows, when they grow, and how they grow. Our seasonal workings for protection, abundance, health, peace, love, and transformation are cued by our local allies as they peak in virtue. In a short time, we end up writing our own materia medica and green grammar which centers the plant people who grow from the same soil we do.

Another exciting aspect of plant priesthood is creating human community through working groups. As you find like-minded folks, you can find creative ways to come together in honor of the green realm, the old deities, the land, the seasons, and stewarding your local area. A bunch of animist plant folk picking up litter at a local park often evolves into something unexpectedly magical.

If you feel called to this work, love it, and find your fulfillment in relationships with the plants and the many inhabitants of the green realm, my hope is that you will continue walking down this ancient track of verdant mysteries. I welcome you to get in touch with me so that we can support one another in the sacredness of relationship in this world and the other.

Please accept my gratitude for reading this book, considering all that is presented here, and maybe even embodying it for yourself. Thank you.

Josh Williams

www.TheGreenArte.com

A GRAMMAR OF THE GREEN ARTE

- Introduction
- A Tea for Every Season
- Hedge Jumping Tea
- Herbal Oil
- Journeying Oil Recipe
- Herbal Salve
- All-Purpose Skin Salve
- Protection
- Invocation Circle Blend`
- Herb-Infused Salt Dough for Vessels and Offerings
- Tinctures

- Wood Wand Balm
- Protective Mantle Wash
- Garland Green
- Cleansing and Clearing Herbs
- Tea Paints
- Preserved Potions
- Ritual Oil
- Divination Medicine
- Entering Trance
- Sacred Plants
- Shrine Tree Opening Ritual
- A Daily Ritual Flow

Introduction

What follows is a small look at some of the pages of my own grammar. I have selected recipes, how-tos, and other pages to show you what this work looks like in practice, and to hopefully inspire you to start your own working book of the green arte.

One of the dangers of grammars and grimoires is our tendency to take them as holy writ. The writings shared here are sacred only to me because they are based on the guidance, teachings, and initiations provided by my own familiar plant spirits. For you, they are inspiration, framework, and map. They are here to lead you to do this work your own way based upon your own relationships with the plants. You can lean on my work for now, but the goal is to invest in the work and own the results rather than following what works in someone else's relationship.

So, as you move through these pages and explore, experiment, and even replicate what I have presented here, I invite you to make plenty of space for your own green arte to develop. See where the recipes take you, then evolve the relationships from there.

As a professional herbalist, I would also like to remind you that what is written here is not intended to treat, cure, diagnose, or prevent any specific illness you may be dealing with. I have tried to share only recipes that are a good fit for most folks, but please do check with a qualified herbalist before adding any of them to your wellness routine.

A tea for every season

Teas are a wonderful way to celebrate the seasons. They are a ritual in and of themselves and invite us into sensual connection with the plants and their medicines. Below are four recipes you can enjoy as the wheel of the year turns.

To make the perfect cup of herbal tea: steep 1 tablespoon of dried blend in 8–10 ounces of steaming-hot water for 9 minutes. Enjoy once comfortably warm.

Parts listed in each recipe are by volume.

Autumn

5 parts Chamomile
1 part dried Apple
1 part Calendula
1 part Basil
1 part Rosehips

Winter

3 parts Holy Basil
2 parts Ginger
1 part Cardamom
1 part Cinnamon
1 part Damiana
1 part Licorice root

Spring

3 parts Lemon Balm
1 part Dandelion root
1 part Cleavers
1 part Chickweed
1 part Shavegrass
1 part Lemon peel
1 part Burdock root

Summer

3 parts Peppermint
1 part Hibiscus
1 part Rose
1 part Hawthorn berry
1 part Nettle
1 part Catnip
1 part Ginkgo

Hedge jumping tea

Enjoy this tea before doing journeywork or traveling to the green realm. Aids in loosening and strengthening the spirit and clarifying visionary capacities.

Steep one tablespoon in 8–10 ounces steaming-hot water for 6 minutes. Strain and enjoy slowly once comfortably warm.

5 parts Peppermint (cooling) or Spearmint (warming)
1 part Brahmi
1 part Hops flowers
1 part California Poppy
1 part Lavender
1 part Rosemary
1 part Mugwort
1 part Fennel seed

Herbal oil

Crafting herbal oils is a simple way to bring the virtues of our plant allies to where we need them most. Infused oils can be used for massage, anointing, body care, baths, or other rituals and are the first step in crafting salves and balms, which we'll cover later on.

Start your herbal oil at the dark moon and allow it to macerate for two weeks. At the full moon, you're done and the oil can be pressed and stored.

In this recipe we do a simple double-extraction using alcohol and oil. This results in a stronger and more aromatic oil with more of the plant's active constituents carrying through.

Here's what you'll need to craft your herbal oil:

- Two clean, dry, glass canning jars with a well-fitting lid
- Sunflower oil
- 120 proof alcohol, such as Everclear (optional)
- Dried herbs
- Cheesecloth
- Paper coffee filters
- Vitamin E oil or Rosemary essential oil
- Labels and glass storage jars

To craft your oil:

- Add dried herbs to one jar. Fill the jar 4/5 of the way full with loosely packed dry herbs.
- Add in 1 tablespoon of 120 proof alcohol, replace the lid, shake well for a minute or two, then leave the jar to sit for 24 hours.
- The next day, open the jar and gently fill with Sunflower oil. Go slowly and allow time for the oil to settle and permeate throughout the herbs. Fill all the way to the top leaving just a hair of room for shaking.
- Replace the lid. Label the jar and place in a warm, dark spot such as a utility cabinet, hot water heater room, or under a sink. Shake once or twice every day to ensure all the herbs are saturated in oil.
- You can leave your oil macerating for up to three months, but two weeks in a warm environment is plenty of time for an excellent infusion.
- Drape cheesecloth over the second jar and gently pour the oil and herb mixture through. Squeeze as much into the jar as you can by wrapping the cheesecloth and twisting it.
- Clean and dry the original jar.
- Fold a paper coffee filter over the rim of the first jar and use the ring or a rubber band to secure it. Gently fill the filter with oil and allow it to slowly drip through, which can take several hours. Once the first pour has been filtered, remove the paper, replace with a new one, and repeat until all of your oil has been filtered.
- Add in two drops of vitamin E or Rosemary essential oil per final ounce of herbal oil as a gentle preservative.
- If your oil has a strong alcohol smell, you can leave the lid off for several hours in a warm room to evaporate it off.

- Store your oil in clearly-labeled glass containers only. Amber colored glass keeps sunlight out and extends the life of your oil. Large batches should be stored in the fridge to prolong their lifespan.

Journeying oil recipe

Craft this oil and apply to pulse points, forehead, and soles of feet before journeywork to help aid in traveling, visioning, and crossing the hedge. The allies we call in for this recipe are:

Mugwort

A celebrated ally who is known to help activate the inner visionary faculties, loosen the spirit, and ease us through the gates into other realms.

Wormwood

Wormwood can help us to quiet the rational mind, activate the fullness of our sensory perception, and still the physical body.

Hops flowers

Famous for beer, Hops is a powerful spirit that has much in common with the virtues of Cannabis. We invoke Hops to this formula in petition of their help with loosening the spirit and opening us up to the subtle ways of the green realm.

Lavender flowers

Lavender is a greatly-honored plant ally the world over. Lavender is called in here to ask their help in quieting the brain, especially the limbic system where our emotional reactivity is rooted, while making us more adaptable to the transformations of journey.

Rose flowers

Rose, often famed as the queen of flowers, is the great guardian of spiritual secrets. Rose protects us with razor-sharp thorns and should be petitioned to help blossom the heart and make one aware of the secrets.

Blend in equal parts using the herbal oil how-to above. You can use this oil as-is, or turn it into a salve or balm using the instructions in the next section.

Herbal salves and balms

Like oils, salves and balms allow us to absorb the virtues of the plants through our skin and apply medicine right where we need it. Salves have a smoother and more oily texture while balms have a denser, drier texture.

You can turn any herbal oil into a salve or balm by following the below method.

Here's what you'll need:

- Beeswax. Locally-sourced wax cut into small beads or pastilles is best.
- Large glass canning jar
- Small sauce pot with two inches of water
- Stovetop
- Coffee stirrers or wooden chopsticks
- Oven mitts
- Containers for your salve or balm
- Labels

To make your salve or balm:

- Bring the water in the pan to a simmer.
- Set the glass canning jar into the water. Ensure that the water doesn't splash up into the jar.
- Here you'll add your herbal oil and beeswax into the jar to melt them down together. To make a softer and oiler salve, I suggest four parts oil to one part wax. For a denser and drier balm, try two parts oil to one part wax. Experiment with different ratios to see what works best for your finished product.
- Once the oil and wax mixture has completely liquefied, use your oven mitts to pour into containers. Allow them to set for several hours before putting on the lids or moving them at all.
- If you don't like the final texture or consistency, you can melt it back down and add more oil or more wax as needed.

- Any essential oils should be added to the liquefied oil and wax blend just before it's poured out into containers. I find six drops of essential oil per ounce a good ratio that's safe for most skin and not overpowering in aroma.
- Salves and balms can be stored in a dark, cool place for several years. Make small batches that you'll get through quickly to avoid having to worry about preservation or storage.

All-purpose skin salve

Craft this nourishing salve to help soothe and strengthen the skin. Great for gardner's hands, feet, or caring for cuticles.

3 parts Calendula
2 part Plantain leaf
1 part Rose flowers
1 part Oregano
1 part Comfrey leaf
1 part Lavender flowers

Protection balm

Apply to pulse points or specific areas of the body when protective energy is needed.

3 parts Holy Basil
2 part Chamomile
2 part St. John's Wort
1 part Angelica root
1 part Hawthorn berries

Invocation circle blend

I love using this fragrant and free-flowing powder to draw circles into which I invoke the plant spirits during rituals, dedications, and workings. You are encouraged to adjust the recipe to include your closest herbal allies, but these herbs can remain as celebrated guides and guardians in the work.

Finely powder in a mortar and pestle or electric spice grinder equal parts of:

Rose flowers
Angelica root
Holy Basil
Elecampane root
St. John's Wort

Measure out the total volume of all powdered herbs and add that same amount of cornmeal or flour.

Blend well with intention and store in a dry glass container away from heat and light.

Herb-infused salt dough

This simple salt dough recipe can be used to craft eco-friendly offerings or vessels for the plant spirits to join you on your shrine. They do melt when wet!

What you'll need:

- Organic flour
- Table salt
- Water
- Powdered or ground herbs of your choosing
- Parchment-lined baking sheet
- Oven pre-heated to 205°F
- Mixing bowl

To make your salt dough:

Combine 2 cups of flour with ½ cup of salt in the mixing bowl. Slowly add in ¾ cup of water taking breaks to knead every ¼ cup. Once all ingredients are combined, knead well, and add in more flour or water as needed to get a nice pliable dough consistency. Add in the herbs.

Sculpt your creations. Anything over about ¾" thick might have a hard time drying and setting, so sticking to ½" thick pieces is ideal.

Once done, place on the paper-lined baking sheet and put into the oven. These generally take around two hours to fully set, but I suggest checking yours every twenty minutes to see if they've become firm to the touch.

Once done, remove from the oven and allow to cool completely before handling. If they feel like they need a bit more time to dry, they can go back in the over or be left out overnight.

Tinctures

Tinctures are a simple way to preserve and work with the medicinal and magical virtues of the plants. I like to begin my tinctures on the dark moon and allow them to macerate as the moon grows in strength and brightness. At the full moon, pressing and bottling tinctures can be part of your ritual observances or just as a way to align to the tides.

When making tinctures, it's crucial that whatever alcohol you choose is around 30%–35% alcohol by volume. Vodka is perfect as are many types of whisky, rum, gin, and brandy.

Here's what you'll need:

- Two glass canning jars
- Dried herbs
- Alcohol
- Large measuring cup
- Cheesecloth
- Paper coffee filters
- Labels and glass dropper bottles

Depending on how much herbal material you are working with, choose a jar that's just over half full when all the herbs are inside. Fill the jar all the way to the top with alcohol leaving just a hair of room for shaking. Label and shake at least once per day. Bringing a tincture crafting into a plant spirit invocation adds a powerful new level of magic and medicine to what's inside. I like to start my tinctures inside the invocation circle, then keep them on my plant spirit shrine during their maceration phase. Jars can be topped with a candle as a way to connect with them each day and put more energy into the process.

After at least two weeks, strain the contents of the jar through cheesecloth draped over a large measuring cup. Affix a paper coffee filter to the other canning jar using the lid or a rubber band, and slowly pour small amounts of the tincture through. The coffee filter can be replaced anew as each pour finished filtering. Once done, pour into glass dropper bottles and label.

Stress tincture formula

This formula helps to calm the mind, easy anxious thinking into more positive spaces, quiet the cortisol response, and relax the body. I like to take half a dropperful up to 5 times per day.

2 parts Holy Basil
2 parts Skullcap
1 part Brahmi
1 part Hawthorn Berries
1 part Catnip
1 part Milky Oats

Journey tincture formula

This potent formula helps with spiritual vision, journeying, and meditation. I like to take 10–15 drops prior to spirit flight.

3 parts Chamomile
1 part California Poppy
1 part Mugwort
1 part Rose
1 part Orange peel

Digestive bitters

I like to take half a dropperful of this aromatic formula to help with many stomach troubles, including gas, bloating, indigestion, or food stagnation.

1 part Chamomile
1 part Angelica root
1 part Fennel seed
1 part Ginger root
1 part Licorice root
1 part Dandelion root

Wood wand balm

Use this waxy balm to hydrate, protect, and seal your wood wand or other wood working tools.
What you'll need:

- Beeswax
- Linseed oil
- Myrrh Gum essential oil
- Pine essential oil

Using the same method as for crafting salves and balms, melt down 1 tablespoon beeswax, 2 tablespoons linseed oil, 6 drops Myrrh essential oil and 6 drops Pine essential oil. Pour into a container and allow to set.

Protective mantle wash

This simple wash adds the protective power of several herbal allies to ritual garb. I like to re-do this wash once per year when the tides turn from dark to bright.
To make your protective wash, brew a strong tea with 1/8 cup of each of the following herbs and enough steaming-hot water to cover them by double:

- Angelica root
- Astragalus root
- St. John's Wort

Steep tea for 30 minutes, then soak your mantle or other cloth. Allow it to air dry. Wash again if needed. Be aware that this tea can stain some materials.

Garland green

Ritual or everyday beaded jewelry can be made from the berries of some of our most cherished plant spirit allies. If you're close to a plant that makes berries, this can be an effective way to carry them with you in ritual or as you journey through life. Most of these berries will crack or split if you try to drill through them once dry, so in this method we work with them while they're perfectly ripe.

Some of the best berries to work with for making beads include Hawthorn, Goji, Rosehips, Rowan, Juniper, and Schisandra.

To craft your garland, string the beads up using a strong embroidery needle and waxed cotton thread just after they've been harvested. The berries should be ripe and supple without being too soft or too easy to squish.

Once they're threaded up, hang them somewhere dry and give them several weeks to fully cure. After that they can be worn around the next, hung on a shrine or tree, used for rituals to mark a circle, or restrung to make more elaborate jewelry.

Cleansing and clearing herbs

Working with our herbal allies to cleanse and clear a space is incredibly effective and is often the easiest way to begin connecting to bioregional plant spirits. Herbs help to purify the atmosphere of energetic static, clear us of distractions and energetic attachments so that we can be more present in rituals, and purify sacred tools and spaces. There are several ways to work with herbs for cleansing and clearing, my favorites being burning, sweeping, and washing.

Dried herbs can be bundled while fresh, given several weeks to dry, then burned to fumigate a space or smoldered on incense charcoals. They can be strewn about a room, petitioned to absorb any negative influences in the space, then ritually swept out the front door, or made into a strong tea which is used to wash floors and walls.

Most cleansing and clearing herbs are evergreen, astringent, and have antiseptic medicinal virtues. A few to consider that might be growing near you include Juniper, Pine, Lavender, Rosemary, St. John's Wort, Angelica, Hyssop, Wormwood, and Sagebrush.

Be mindful of plants that are sacred to the indigenous people of your area and of methods for cleansing and clearing that are part of closed practices. Avoid plant allies like Sage, Sweetgrass, and Palo Santo to ensure that the folks who have ancient ties to these plants have continued access to them and that we don't support poaching threatened plants from delicate bioregions.

Tea paints

Strong herbal teas can be made and used as watercolors for spirit houses, magical workings, or creative communications with the plant spirits. Some of the dried herbs that make the most vibrant paint colors include: Butterfly Pea Flower, Elder Berries, Cinnamon Sticks, Allspice Berries, Juniper Berries, Nettle, Hawthorn Berries, Turmeric Root, Hibiscus Flowers, and Alfalfa.

To make the strongest pigment, try pouring steaming-hot water to just above the top of the dried herbs. Cover, and allow them to steep for several hours or overnight. I like to use little two-ounce canning jars for this and find it makes the perfect amount of paint for a group of people to play with. You can strain the herbs from the water or leave them settled in the bottom. Strained tea paints can be refrigerated for several days before they start to turn.

Potions

Potions are created in ritual by invoking the plant spirit or spirits involved into the finished potion, and asking for the blessings of the plants. Potions can be taken as a single 'shot' or sipped on in measured doses over a specific amount of time. They do have an expiry and should be kept refrigerated, so bear that in mind when working this method of magic. I like potions for situations where bringing a more ritually-made medicine into the actual body is called for. As always, ensure that the herbs you work with are safe for consumption and that the whole process is handled with good food safety measures.

I use a traditional oxymel to craft my potions and love the sweet and tangy kick they give, plus their super effective extraction of the herbs themselves. Here's what you'll need to make your potion:

- Raw, local, wild honey (substitute agave if needed)
- Apple cider vinegar
- Dried herbs
- Parchment or wax paper
- Glass canning jar with lid. This jar should be halfway full when all your dried herbs are placed inside.

- Small, aesthetic glass bottle to store your potion. The dosing for these is about 1 ounce, so keep that in mind. Larger bottles can be used if they contain several doses of the potion.
- Labels and decorations for the bottles as desired

To craft your potion, consider starting at the dark moon in a ritual setting with the presence of the plant allies, elder gods, and ancestors joining you.

- Fill your glass canning jar ¼ full of dried herbs
- Top off with an even balance of honey and apple cider vinegar leaving as little room at the top as possible.
- Clean the jar of any honey and make sure the threads and lid are especially clean so they don't get stuck together.
- Place a double-layer of paper over the mouth of the jar, then put the lid on. This is to prevent the acidic vinegar from coming into contact with the metal lid. Plastic wrap can also be used here if paper isn't available.
- Label what's inside and make a place for your potion on a medicine altar or plant spirit shrine.
- Take time to connect with the magic happening within at least once per day, and add energy and movement by shaking for 30–60 seconds.
- At the two-week mark, ideally on the full of the moon, strain the contents through fine cheesecloth, twice if needed, and bottle up with labels.
- Potions made in this manner are shelf stable for up to six months. I keep mine in the refrigerator just to be safe. Once opened, they should be consumed within a few days and kept cold.

Again, I would suggest no more than one ounce as a single dose. These potions are strong, and the acidity of the vinegar can be intense for some people. I was able to find some lovely three-ounce glass bottles in a vintage shape that I like to use. This provides three doses of potion over three days and can be paired with a candle or incense for a daily ritual experience.

Vitality potion

To nourish the body and support inner strength.

Equal parts
Nettle leaf
Red Clover blossoms
Milky Oats
A pinch of Cinnamon

Ritual potion

Work with this potion before rituals, magic, or journeywork.

2 parts Holy Basil
1 part Hyssop
1 part Chamomile
1 part Rose flowers
1 part Angelica root

Sacred breath potion

To help deepen the breath, support the respiratory system, cleanse and detox the lungs, and connect breathing to the mind.

1 part Elecampane root
1 part Mullein flowers
1 part Lavender flowers
1 part Astragalus root
and a small pinch of Cardamom seeds

Ritual oil

Craft this fragrant oil for use in all your plant spirit ritual workings. Can be used to anoint the body, candles, statues, spaces, and more.
   Using the infused oil how-to provided earlier, make your oil with:

1 part Lavender flowers
1 part Juniper berries
1 part Cedar or Pine needles

1 part Rose flowers
1 part Astragalus root
1 part Hops flowers (Cannabis flowers can also be used but may be more intoxicating)
1 part Chamomile flowers
1 part Holy Basil
1 part St. John's Wort

Divination allies

Here are a few various recipes I love to work with when doing divinations.

Divination tea

3 parts Lemon Balm
1 part Hops flowers
1 part California Poppy
1 part Licorice root
1 part Rose flowers
1 part Holy Basil

Divination incense

Combine equal parts of all and burn on an incense charcoal in an urn.

Rose
Chamomile
Angelica root
Hops
Lavender

Divination oil

Anoint pulse points before divinations. Combine equal parts when crafting an infused oil.

Rosemary
Rose
Lavender

Hops
Chamomile

Entering trance

There are countless effective ways to drop into light or heavy trance states for journeywork, spirit flight, meditation, and ritual. Here are a few of my favorites.

Bardic method

This method is inspired by a technique used by the Irish bards to help facilitate poetic inspiration. It works by using the peripheral nervous system to quiet the senses and bring vividness to the inner vision.

Lie on your back in ritual space, surrounded by a sacred grove. Place a heavy book or other object on the center of your chest, no more than about three to five pounds. The eyes can be covered with a light cloth to help further induce the trance state. Focus on your breathing and feel yourself drop in. If you experience any difficulty in breathing, lighten the weight or try another method.

Labyrinth

Troy-town labyrinths or other patterns can be traced with the finger or the eyes to help facilitate trance induction. A simple carved maze in clay or wood can be taken with the tip of the finger to help quiet the senses and alter the consciousness, or a large print of a maze can be traced with the eyes.

Box breathing

Slow, gentle, deep, and relaxed breathing patterns can be followed while gazing at a tree or your shrine to help drop you into a trance state. Find a count that works for your body and use that same count for the inhale, hold, exhale, and hold to form a box pattern in your breathing. Once in trance, you can release the breath to its usual rhythm and continue on with your work.

Shrine tree opening ritual

As mentioned in the book, I keep the image of a tree on my shrine to represent the plant spirits *all* and to act as a focal point for my spirit journeys. This tree is decorated to reflect the energies of the seasons and is the central axis for much of my home shrine work.

Opening the tree shrine is a way to establish a potent flow of vital force through it so that it can work as a crossroads of liminality in your sacred space. This simple ritual helps connect your tree to the world tree, and you to your tree.

- Place one hand at the base of the tree symbol and the other hand at the top.
- Imagine a stream of vital force, energy, light, or power surging between your palms and through the tree.
- Once you feel the tree icon has been saturated with power, envision the world tree and align it with your icon so that they overlap. This can be done with eyes open or closed, whichever is easiest for you.
- Experience the tree icon having energetic roots that reach deep into the land below you and an energetic canopy that reaches up high into the sky above you.
- Place the tree on your shrine and see it as a meeting point between you and the green realm.

A daily ritual flow

Establishing a consistent ritual connection to the plant spirits and other denizens of the green arte is a great way to build a strong foundation on which to build the work. As you show up time and time again, the spirits are better able to work with you to create a deep relationship and strong spiritual spaces. The following ritual flow is simple and leaves a great deal of room for personalization should you want to change anything. As-is, this flow is how I teach students to sit with a single plant ally every day as they cultivate new magico-medicinal working relationships in the green realm. Here, these same steps are also applied to cultivating a relationship with the deities, ancestors, and spirits of place. As always, make adjustments where needed and where you're guided to.

- Set the Altar
  Begin every ritual by creating sacred space. If you have a permanent altar to the spirits of the green arte, you may need to do very little. If you don't have something permanent, this step is an invitation to carve out some space in your physical world for the plant spirits, deities, ancestors, and spirits of place to settle in and join with you in your work.
- Invocation
  The invocation process is one of creating intentional space for the spirits to join you, of making a conscious effort to call them in and make them welcome, and in changing your own internal atmosphere to one that is more aware of their sometimes subtle ways of being.

  I like to make an organic, spontaneous invocation to whomever I wish to join me, one at a time. I might invite *the plant spirits all*, specific individual plant spirits I work with or am getting to know, my deities, my good and blessed ancestors, and the spirits of place who share their space with me in peace and plenty. Don't overthink this. Instead, feel your way through it. Say what feels good inside you and that kindles the beacon of light which really attracts the spirits.
- Sharing Breath
  Spend a few minutes simply sharing in the sacred act of breath with your allies; offer your exhalation as a gift, receive the gifts of the green realm through your inhalation. This is a powerful part of our plant spirit work and one that can lead us to many surprising places.
- Make Offerings
  This is your opportunity to participate daily in the act of sacred reciprocity. It is here that we express our gratitude and love for our allies while also ensuring that we pay our debts and return the energies which have been sent to us so that the endless cycle continues without hindrance. Your offerings can be as simple or grandiose as you like. Libations of clean water, liquor, or wine, pinches of rice charged with your energy, words or songs of praise, botanical incense, beeswax candles, and so on are all appropriate daily offerings. I tend to focus on lighting incense and wafting the smoke in the direction of each of my allies in turn after lighting candles on each of their shrine areas. The candles burn, the incense rises, and I spend just a few minutes breathing, connecting, and being receptive to my sacred relationships.

- Listen and Commune
  We have now invoked the spirits, entered into magical breath sharing with them, and gifted them. From here the most powerful thing we can do is simply listen. Be as fully present in the moment and in the space you've created as possible. Listen from *everywhere*. Imagine that everything that comes up for you in this space is meaningful and allow it to fully unfold without judgment or restriction.

  This is also a time when you can commune directly with any plant spirits you're sitting with. Petitions, praises, gratitudes, or shares can all be offered here in a dynamic conversation.
- Embodiment and Journaling
  Honor what you receive no matter how small it may seem or how much 'your own voice' you may feel it is. Write your experiences down in a journal or repeat them to anchor them in your being.
- Venturing Out
  Carry the experience, blessing, wisdom, and guidance of this ritual with you out into your life. Look forward to sitting with the verdant spirits again tomorrow!

STAY CONNECTED

I hope that you enjoyed this book and whatever journey it may have taken you on. If you found the material interesting, I would love to hear from you. At this moment I am quite active on social media and have several online courses I'd love for you to join me on in addition to many classes on my YouTube channel.

I hope to connect with you soon!

Josh Williams

www.TheGreenArte.com
Instagram & YouTube: @TheGreenArte

REFERENCES AND RESOURCES

Harvey, Graham. *Animism, Respecting the Living World.* Columbia University Press, 2005.
Wall-Kimmerer, Robin. *Braiding Sweetgrass.* Milkweed Editions, 2014.
Matthews, John. *Quest for The Green Man.* Quest Books, 2001.
O'Brien, Lora. *Irish Witchcraft.* 2nd Ed. Eel & Otter Press, 2020.
Daimler, Morgan. *Fairycraft.* John Hunt Publishing Ltd., 2015.
Evans-Wentz, W.Y. *The Faery-Faith in Celtic Countries.* Citadel Press, 1994.
Beyerl, Paul. *Master Book of Herbalism.* Phoenix Publishing Inc., 1984.
Beyerl, Paul. *A Compendium of Herbal Magick.* Phoenix Publishing Inc., 1998.
Thistleton-Dyer, T.F. *The Mythic & Magical Folklore of Plants.* Lulu, 2008.
Folkard, Richard. *Plant Lore, Legends, and Lyrics.* Forgotten Books, 2012.

Pollington, Stephen. *Leechcraft: Early English Charms, Plant-Lore, and Healing*. Anglo-Saxon Books, 2000.
Williams, Josh. *Spiritual Herbalism: The Magic and Medicine of the Plants*. Aeon Books, 2022
Lecouteux, Claude. *The Return of the Dead*. Inner Traditions, 2009.
Lecouteux, Claude. *Demons and Spirits of the Land*. Inner Traditions, 2015.
Yunkaporta, Tyson. *Sand Talk*. HarperOne, 2021.
Curran, Dr. Bob. *Walking with The Green Man*. Red Wheel/Weiser, 2007.
Tierra, Michael. *Planetary Herbology*. Lotus Press, 1992.
Carmichael, Alexander. *Carmina Gadelica*. Floris Books, 1994.
Horne, Roger J. *Folk Witchcraft*. Independently Published, 2019.
Penczak, Christopher. *The Plant Spirit Familiar*. Copper Cauldron Publishing, 2011.
Montgomery, Pam. *Plant Spirit Healing*. Bear & Co., 2008.
Darrell, Nikki. *Conversations with Plants*. Aeon Books, 2020.
Waller, Pip & Wells, Lucy. *Touched by Nature*. Aeon Books, 2019.
Schulke, Daniel. *Thirteen Pathways of Occult Herbalism*. Three Hands Press, 2017.
Artisson, Robin. *An Carow Gwyn*. Independently Published, 2019.
Rowan Laurie, Erynn. *Ogam: Weaving Word Wisdom*. Megalithica Books, 2007.

INDEX

after death, 82–83. *See also* ancestral veneration
all-purpose skin salve, 240
amulets, 180. *See also* plant spirit magic
ancestors
    charm to honor, 219
    lore, 25, 69
    types of, 82
ancestral veneration, 81
    ancient symbol associated with green man, 82
    after death, 82–83
    offerings to dead, 83–84
    types of ancestors, 82
ancient tracks, 2, 59
    land and, 200–201
    map of, 3
animal spirits, 72–73
animism, 15–16, 55–56, 156
    and arte, 64
    code of anti-ethics and, 200
animist cosmology, 61
Ashvattha, 29
Assyrian Moon Tree, 29–30
autumn fête, 94–96. *See also* sacred calendars

balm, 181. *See also* plant spirit magic
  protection, 240
  wood wand, 244
Bardic method, 250
baths and washes, 179. *See also* plant spirit magic
being a person, 15
bells, 168. *See also* tools of arte
bowl, 163–164. *See also* tools of arte
box breathing, 250
breath, 41, 43
  breathing, 42
  fight-or-flight system, 42
  plant respiration, 41
  reciprocity, 42–43
  ritual breathing, 43
  stomata, 41
  tree speed, 42
  vital force, 46
breathing, 42, 48
  box, 250
  green, 56
bright solstice, 93–94. *See also* sacred calendars

candles, 178–179, 211. *See also* plant spirit magic
canopy, 31, 47–48. *See also* world tree symbol
casting staves, 194. *See also* divination
Celtic lore, 200–201
charms, 218–219
chlorophyll, 37–38
  breathing green, 38, 40
  field of green, 38
  green mantle, 38–39, 40
  receiving green, 40
cleansing, 189
  and clearing herbs, 245
cledonism technique, 194–195. *See also* divination
collective healing, 155. *See also* plant medicine
communicating with plants, 55
constitutional medicine, 156. *See also* plant medicine

crown pool, 47

daily ritual flow, 251–253
dance of deities, 66–69. *See also* deities, old
dark solstice, 89–90. *See also* sacred calendars
dedication. *See* plant spirit dedications
  9-day, 127
  3-day, 125–126
  29-day lunar cycle, 125
deities, old, 63
  animism and arte, 64
  dance of, 66–69
  Great Green God/The Green Man, 64–65
  Land Goddess, 66
  opening vessels for, 215
  ways to connect with, 69–70
devocation, 191
digestive bitters, 243
divination, 193
  allies, 249–250
  casting staves, 194
  cledonism technique, 194–195
  communing with Green Man, 194
  exploration of tree, 194
  guidance of land, 195
  incense, 249
  nature's response, 194–195
  Ogham, 196–197
  oil, 249–250
  omens, 196
  tea, 249
  tools, 168
  winds, 195–196
doctrine of signatures, 170
dry respiratory herbs, 157–158. *See also* plant medicine

energetic herbalism, 157. *See also* plant medicine
energetics, 156–158
energy flow and healing work, 48–50
equinoxes, 96. *See also* sacred calendars

INDEX 261

Faery tales. *See* lore
familiar green spirit, 133
    connection between us and plant spirit, 134
fight-or-flight system, 42
flame, 211
flow of life, 31–32. *See also* world tree symbol
foison, 184. *See also* shared meal
folktales. *See* lore
full moon, 98. *See also* lunar tides
    rite, 99–103

garland, 86. *See also* sacred calendars
    green, 244–245
good folk/faery, 73–74
grammar, 59, 233, 234
Great Green God. *See* Green Man
green
    breathing, 56
    gnosis, 26
    grammar, 59–60
    Green God, 1
    mantle, 38–39, 40. *See also* chlorophyll
    mystery, 4
Green Arte, The, 4, 7, 71, 217
Green Man, 64–65. *See also* deities, old
    ancient symbol associated with, 82
    charm to invoke, 218
    communing with, 194
green realm, 33
    entering, 35
    life energy, 34
    metabolism, 33–34
    plant spirits, 34
    sacred cycle of reciprocity, 34
    sacred place, 34
    spirit flight, 34
green ritual, 187
    cleansing, 189
    devocation, 191
    invocations and offerings, 190
    marking the space, 188
    raising the hedge, 190
    reciting petition to spirits, 188–189
    releasing the hedge, 191
    shared meal, 191
    steps of ritual flow, 188
    working with plant spirit, 190
grimoire, 59, 234
growing plant, 180–181. *See also* plant spirit magic
guidance of land, 195. *See also* divination

healing, 48–50, 137
    collective, 155
    energetic herbalism, 157
    spiritual herbalism, 160
heart, 225–226
    pool, 47
    wild within, 226–227
hedge, 11
    jumping tea, 236
    releasing the, 191
hedge, raising the, 105, 107–108, 190
    allies of protection, 107
    charm to, 218
    deflecting negative energies, 107
    finding peace and safety, 106
    protection, 106
hedgerow, 105
hedgewalker, 11–13
    hedge, 11
    nature of, 13
    wise person, 11–12
herb
    dry respiratory, 157–158
    -infused salt dough, 241
    oils, 236–238
    salves and balms, 239–240
herbalism, 160. *See also* plant medicine
    energetic, 157
    spiritual, 158
hops flowers, 238
humoural medicine, 156. *See also* plant medicine

icons. *See* plant spirit vessels
incense
    and bundles, 178
    urn, 165–166
initiation, 9, 10, 158–159
inner vision, 51
invocation, 1–2, 100, 101, 102, 117
    circle blend, 240–241
    and offerings, 190

journeying oil recipe, 238–239
journey tincture formula, 243

keep, the, 223–224
kith and kin, 61
    ancestors, 81–84
    old deities of arte, 63–70
    relationships, 62
    spirits of nature, 71–75

labyrinths, 250
Lady of the Land, 95. *See also* sacred calendars
land and ancient tracks, 200–201
Land Goddess, 66. *See also* deities, old
language of plants, 54–55
lavender flowers, 238
legends. *See* lore
life cycle of tree, 31. *See also* world tree symbol
life energy, 34
life, flow of, 31–32. *See also* world tree symbol
lore, 25–27, 170
    Celtic, 200–201
Lughnasadh, 94. *See also* sacred calendars
lunar tides, 97
    full moon, 98
    full moon rite, 99–103
    invocation, 100, 101, 102
    moon phases, 98
    waning moon, 98–99
    waxing moon, 98

magic, 173. *See also* plant spirit magic
mantle, 39, 167. *See also* tools of arte
map to green realm, 109, 111–112
    gateway gods, 115
    journey to green realm, 112–114
    magic and medicine from roots, 115
    plant spirit liminality, 110
    tree at crossroads, 110
    wortriding, 114
material medica, 170–172
medicine, 169–172
    dreams, 56–57
metal, 164, 202. *See also* tools of arte
middle world, 31
moon phases, 98. *See also* lunar tides
mortar and pestle, 162–163. *See also* tools of arte
mugwort, 238
Mullein (*Verbascum thapsus*), 157
mysteries, 10
myths. *See* lore

nature's response, 194–195. *See also* divination
9-day dedication, 127

offering, 212–213
    blend, 167
    bowl, 166–167
    to dead, 83–84
Ogham, 196–197. *See also* divination
oils and balms, 181. *See also* plant spirit magic
omens, 196. *See also* divination
otherworld, 30

personhood, 18–19, 21
petition, 151, 219
    and prayers, 213
    relationship, 152
    rituals, 151–152
    to spirits, 188–189
    on the path, 220
    ways to asking help, 152–153

plant
    as living bridge, 23
    mysteries, 170
    priesthood, 229–232
    respiration, 41
    spirit work, 8
    taboos, 203–204
    tribes and clans, 22
    and world, 22
plant medicine, 155
    animism, 156
    collective healing, 155
    constitutional or *humoural* medicine, 156
    dry respiratory herbs, 157–158
    energetic herbalism, 157
    energetics, 156–158
    giving medicine, 159–160
    herbalism, 160
    initiation, 158–159
    spiritual herbalism, 158
plant spirit communication, 53
    animism, 55–56
    communicating with plants, 55
    green breathing, 56
    language of plants, 54–55
    medicine dreams, 56–57
    sacred connection point, 55
plant spirit dedications, 123
    beginning ritual, 124
    9-day dedication, 127
    paths to work, 124
    rituals *dedications*, 124
    3-day dedication, 125–126
    29-day lunar cycle dedication, 125
    29-lunar cycle dedication, 127–131
plant spirit magic, 173
    amulets, 180
    baths and washes, 179
    candles, 178–179
    expressions of, 177
    growing plant, 180–181
    incense and bundles, 178
    key steps, 174
    making magic, 175

    oils and balms, 181
    potions, 182
    powders, 180
    ritual framework, 175–176
    sachets, 177–178
    tinctures, 181–182
plant spirits, 21, 34
    developing spirit vision, 26
    green gnosis, 26
    lore, 25–27
    plant as living bridge, 23
    plant tribes and clans, 22
    working with, 22, 190
plant spirit shrines, 139
    food alternate offerings, 142
    offerings, 141
    realm of Faery and green realm, 141
    ritual of opening, 142–143
    uses for, 140
plant spirits, invoking, 117
    full invocation and medicine ritual, 121–122
    invocation ritual, 118–120
plant spirit vessels, 145
    for creative inspiration, 146–147
    opening the vessel, 148–149
potion, 182, 246–247. *See also* plant spirit magic
    sacred breath, 248
    vitality, 248
powders, 180. *See also* plant spirit magic
priests of plants. *See* plant—priesthood
primordial forest, 7
Privet (*Ligustrum vulgare*), 106
protection balm, 240
protective mantle wash, 244

reciprocal breath, 42–43
relationships of rightness, 15
    animism, 15–16
    being a person, 15
    personhood, 18–19, 21
    respect, 17–18
respect, 17–18

ritual
- breathing, 43
- cup and plate, 166
- cycles, 86
- oil, 248–249
- potion, 248
- shrine tree opening ritual, 251
- writing rituals of rightness, 220–221

roots of living tree, 30. *See also* world tree symbol
rose flowers, 238–239

sachets, 177–178. *See also* plant spirit magic
sacred breath potion, 248
sacred calendars, 85
- autumn fête, 94–96
- bright solstice, 93–94
- dark solstice, 89–90
- equinoxes, 96
- garland, 86
- Lady of the Land, 95
- Lughnasadh, 94
- ritual cycles, 86
- Samhuinn, 86
- seasons and festivals, 86
- spring fête, 90–92
- summer fête, 92–93
- timing, 96
- winter fête, 86–89

sacred circles, 77–79
sacred color, 37. *See also* chlorophyll
sacred connection point, 55
sacred cycle of reciprocity, 34
sacred fires, 135
- of possession, 136
- ritual fires, 137

sacred place, 34
sacred spaces, 77–79
- in animist traditions, 72
- tending to, 209–210

sacred symbolism, 212
Samhuinn, 86. *See also* sacred calendars
seasons and festivals, 86. *See also* sacred calendars
sewing kit, 165. *See also* tools of arte

shared meal, 183, 191
foison, 184
- rite to honor someone, 185–186
- taboos, 202–203
- things needed for, 184–185
- ways to offer, 184

shrine and grove tending, 209
- flame, 211
- offerings, 212–213
- opening vessels for deities, 215
- petitions and prayers, 213
- sacred symbolism, 212
- seasonal reflections, 211
- setting up shrine, 210–211
- taboos, 214
- tending to sacred space, 209–210

shrine tree opening ritual, 251
skin salve, all-purpose, 240
sorcery, 217
sounds, 168. *See also* tools of arte
sovereignty, 207
spirit
- houses. *See* plant spirit vessels
- of place, 72
- vision, 26
- world, 33

spirit flight, 34, 109
- gateway gods, 115
- journey to green realm, 112–114
- magic and medicine from roots, 115
- map, 111–112
- plant spirit liminality, 110
- tree at crossroads, 110
- wortriding, 114

spirits of nature, 71
- animal spirits, 72–73
- *good folk*/faery, 73–74
- observing land and inhabitants, 75
- spirits of place, 72

spiritual herbalism, 158. *See also* plant medicine
spring fête, 90–92. *See also* sacred calendars
stewardship, 205–207
stomata, 41

stress tincture formula, 243
summer fête, 92–93. *See also* sacred calendars
symbolism, 29

taboos, 199
  calling by name, 201–202
  Celtic lore, 200–201
  code of anti-ethics and animism, 200
  food, 202–203
  land and ancient tracks, 200–201
  metals, 202
  plant taboos, 203–204
  regarding shrine tending, 214
tea paints, 246
teas, 235–236
therapeutic, intentional touch, 50–51
3-day dedication, 125–126. *See also* plant spirit dedications
tinctures, 50, 181–182, 242. *See also* plant spirit magic
  journey tincture formula, 243
  making, 120
  stress tincture formula, 243
tools of arte, 161
  bells, 168
  divination tools, 168
  incense urn, 165–166
  mantle, 167
  metal, 164
  mortar and pestle, 162–163
  offering blend, 167
  offering bowl, 166–167
  ritual cup and plate, 166
  sewing kit, 165
  sounds, 168
  verdigris blade, 164–165
  vessel, 163–164
  wand, 163
trance, entering, 250
  Bardic method, 250
  box breathing, 250
  labyrinths, 250
tree
  exploration of, 194

life cycle of, 31
roots of living, 30
speed, 42
trunk, 30–31. *See also* world tree symbol
29-day lunar cycle dedication, 125
29-lunar cycle dedication, 127. *See also* plant spirit dedications
  dark moon, 130–131
  day one, 128–129
  full moon, 129–130
  preparation, 127–128

universe, 61

verdigris blade, 164–165. *See also* tools of arte
vessel, 146, 163–164. *See also* plant spirit vessel; tools of arte
  crafting plant spirit, 140, 146
  for deities, 215
vision, 51
vital force, 45
  breath, 46
  breathing, 48
  canopy, 47–48
  crown pool, 47
  exercise for energy flow, 48–50
  heart pool, 47
  inner vision, 51
  meditation using world tree symbol, 46
  within physical bodies, 46
  plants, 52
  therapeutic, intentional touch, 50–51
  vision, 51
vitality potion, 248

wand, 163. *See also* tools of arte
waning moon, 98–99. *See also* lunar tides
winds, 195–196. *See also* divination
winter fête, 86–89. *See also* sacred calendars
wood wand balm, 244

world of spirit, 33
world tree symbol, 29
    canopy, 31
    flow of life, 31–32
    gateway, 32
    journey, 32
    life cycle of tree, 31
    roots of living tree, 30
    trunk, 30–31
wormwood, 238

Yggdrasil, 29

Printed by Printforce, United Kingdom